Vet School Survival Gui

Notes From A Back Row Student

By

Dean W. Scott, DVM

Dedicated to other survivors of vet school,

specifically my wife, Sue, and

daughters, Heather and Caitlin

"Humor heightens our sense of survival

and preserves our sanity."

\- Charlie Chaplin

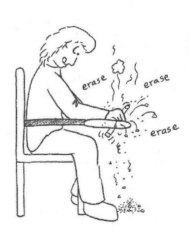

Introduction

Much has changed since I was in veterinary school. Much hasn't. Which is why I think the need for this book is still relevant. So much more is known now about the stresses the veterinary community faces starting as early as the pre-vet phase. When people say to me, "I hear it's hard to get into vet school," I reply, "True, but it's even harder to get out. Wanna see my scars?" I ascribe to the band-aid theory of vet school. That is, you can get through it fast or slow, but either way, it's going to hurt.

I knew veterinary school would be difficult academically, but what I didn't anticipate were some of the other obstacles. Consider the oxymorons: "faculty support" and "student services". Upon entering vet school, I quickly learned it is akin to a circus act, where you are the lion being told to jump through a series of hoops. When you do, this is what you get: "Good. Now a little higher." And when you do that, you hear, "Now let's set the hoops on fire." And this goes on in ever-increasing levels of difficulty.

Under this kind of environment everyone has to have a way to release the stress, hopefully in productive avenues. I coped by identifying stresses and trying to find something humorous in them. This book started as a Top 10 List of Veterinary School Stresses and I quickly realized there were way more than ten!

It may not seem like it now, but this book is probably the most important one you will ever have. Because this book is the closest you'll ever get to understanding what happens in vet school and how to deal with it. Sure, it's done, ultimately, for the laughs, but I think if you look closely enough you'll see it's a pretty good primer for school as well. It's particularly useful for current students as they can check each stress off as they occur. This book is also the only place that will acknowledge the shared experience and adversity that binds this profession together.

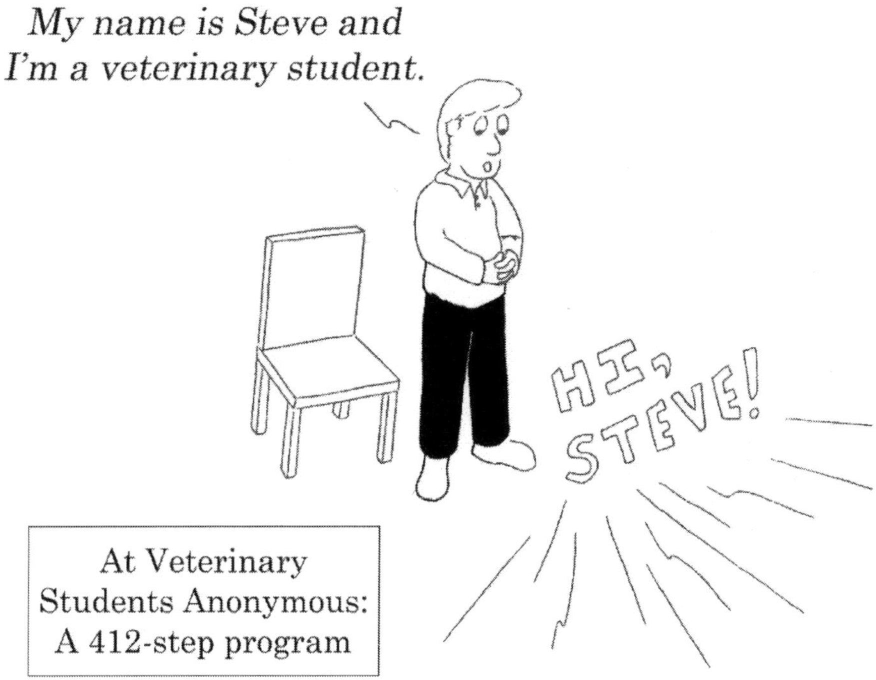

At Veterinary Students Anonymous: A 412-step program

<u>The Top 1,000 Vet School Stresses</u>

Professor shows up to lecture again.

Getting "those" looks from faculty.

Lecture slides shown at the pace of motion pictures.

Not having exact change for your caffeine fix.

Classmates who say, "I understand."

Being told something is obvious or classical
when you're clueless.

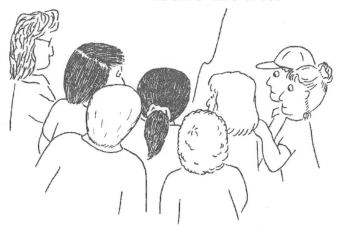

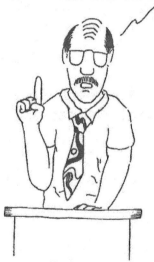

Lectures that should be given with subtitles

No one else shows up to the stress workshop.

Major research person pretends to give you
useful information.

Not being able to concentrate on newspaper
content due to lecturer nattering on.

Being academically impotent, you can't
seem to get your grades up.

Finding notes in your writing that you don't recognize.

You suffer from caffeinemia.

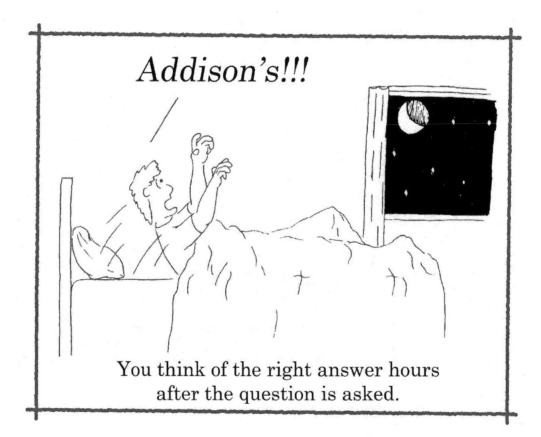

You think of the right answer hours
after the question is asked.

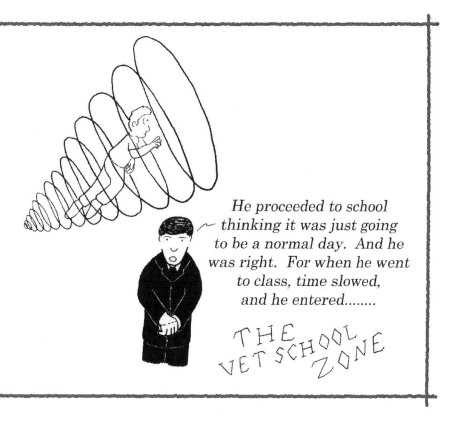

He proceeded to school
thinking it was just going
to be a normal day. And he
was right. For when he went
to class, time slowed,
and he entered........

THE
VET SCHOOL
ZONE

Faculty point and laugh in your direction.

Finding out Lassie was male.

The voices in your head go away and you feel
like you've lost your best friend.

Professors who, as a demonstration, imitate signs
of a fatal disease without following through.

Classmates who say,
"Oh, I could have done better than an A minus."

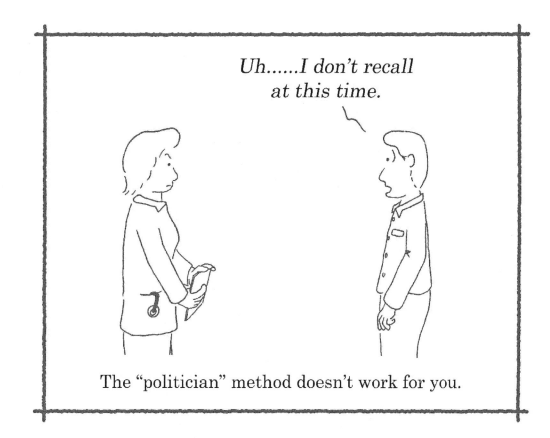

You're given Virtual Reality goggles,
because the curriculum is so unreal.

Classmates who say you should get counseling.

People who feel it necessary to remind you that
"finals are next week".

Complete strangers walk up to you and say
you should get counseling.

Walking halfway to school and realizing that
you forgot your car.

You overdose on toxicology.

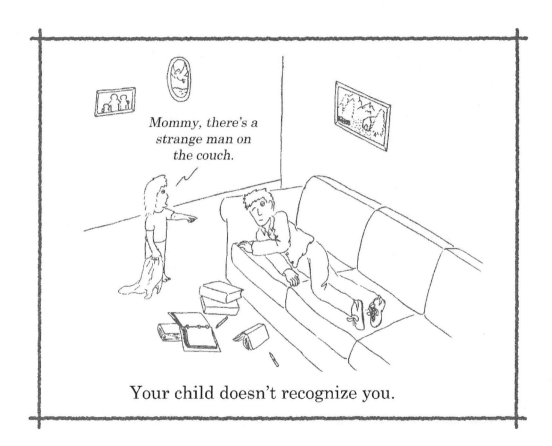

Your child doesn't recognize you.

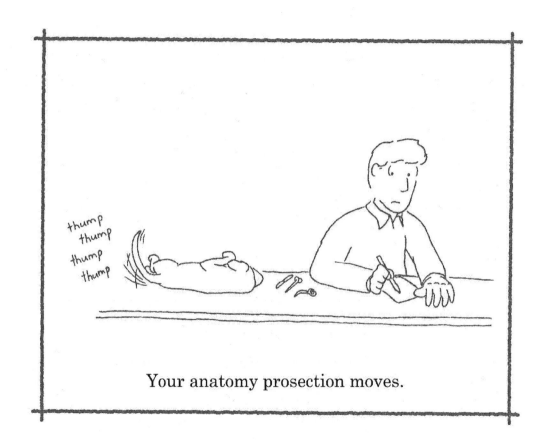

Your anatomy prosection moves.

Knowing you could have done better on an exam
if you had guessed.

Having the concentration differential of the renal tubule
explained one more time and still not getting it.

Discovering your dream about the vet school
burning down was (sigh) just a dream.

Not having any more reasons to procrastinate
on studying.

You lose your watch in the cow you're palpating.

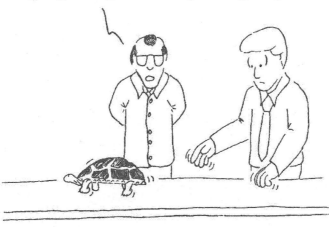

Questions on the exam that were not on any
old class exams you have.

Being recognized by the Dean, but not in a good way.

Discovering that the *Small Animal Medicine* Vols. 1–3
that you just bought for $800
are on sale at WalMart for $100.

Using the ATM to withdraw money
and having it laugh at you.

First year.

Your email notification tune is *Taps*.

Professors who use the words "oral" and "exam"
in the same sentence.

Clueless people who say,
"You must be so excited to be in vet school!"

Someone pinches you and when you wake up
you find out that the last three years of vet school
were just a really, really, really bad dream.

Scantron requiring a #3 pencil.

You stop to think but forget to start again.

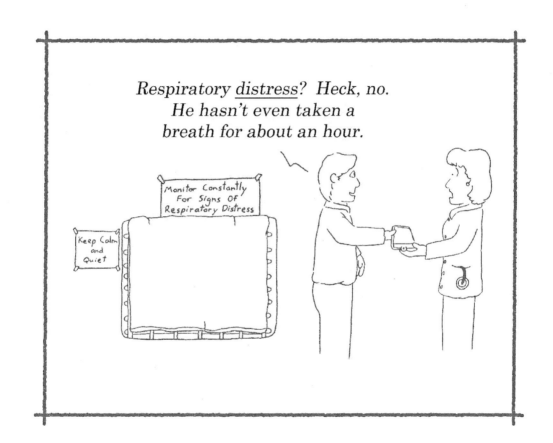

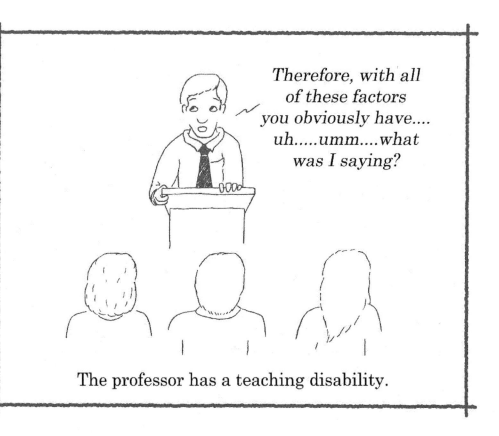

The professor has a teaching disability.

Getting a question correct in rounds and
wondering why the heavens fail to open up
with angels singing, "Hallelujah!".

After you bomb an exam because you studied the notes
rather than the old tests, your classmate, who aced the
exam thanks you for lending the old tests to her.

Inadvertently becoming an intermediate host.

Hare Krishnas cunningly disguised as faculty members
try to recruit you into academia.

You listen to your relaxation tapes on high speed.

Getting good news/bad news from the Student Affairs Committee: the good news is that you'll have abundant free time starting next quarter.

Really old vet says, "I don't envy you having to learn so much new information."

Professors who giggle while grading your exam.

You realize during cardiology just how long it's been since you've had a palpable thrill.

Antacid tablets become your sole source of nutrition.

A classmate gets a gold star on his quiz and you don't.

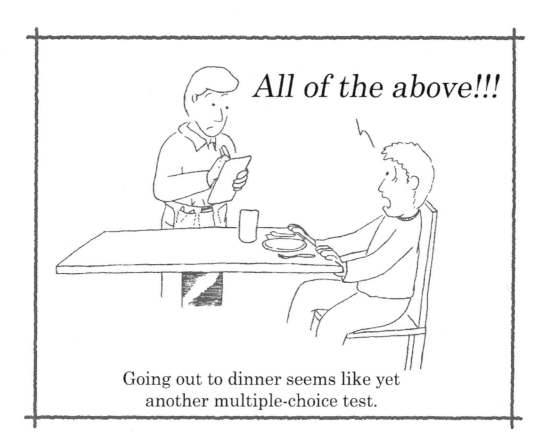

Going out to dinner seems like yet another multiple-choice test.

Getting deathly ill over vacation only to recover just in time for the new quarter.

A previous high school classmate pulls up next to your Nissan Versa in a BMW and asks, "Do you have any Grey Poupon?"

Your significant other doesn't recognize you.

Finally showing up on time for class and then realizing it's a holiday.

You no longer brush your teeth, you float them.

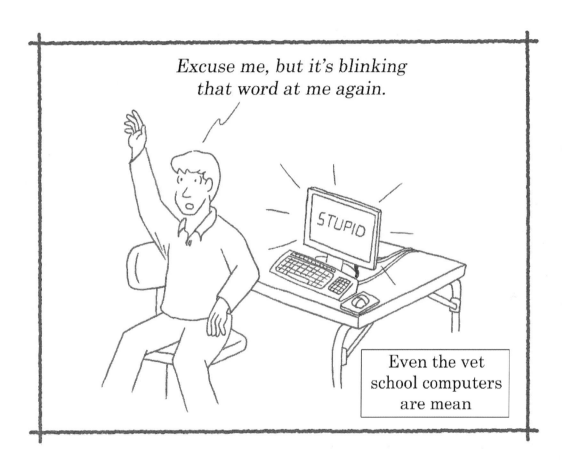

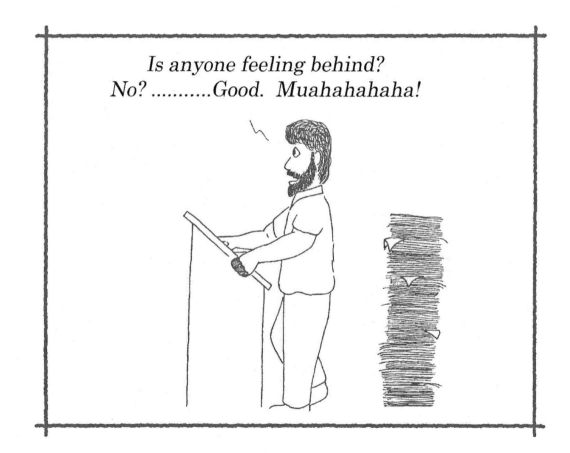

You start looking like your class picture.

You don't recognize this person who insists they're your significant other.

You can't experience a normal conversation with non-vet school people.

A person in the class ahead of you is suddenly in the class behind you.

Three days have passed and you can't recall whether or not you've slept.

Natural light makes you squint.

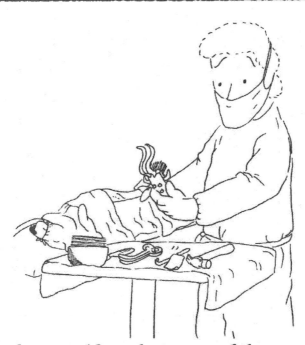

You have no idea what some of the
instruments in your surgery pack are for.

Time-wasting sensitivity workshops
that don't do a bit of good since you have enough
damn sensitivity to last a lifetime!

Your washing machine breaks down because you used it to
wash both your surgery linens and instruments.

Classes that require you to review previous classes.

Surgery videos with the same running time as the
extended versions of *Lord of the Rings*.

You no longer urinate. You coffeenate.

You take the "Don't Walk" signs personally.

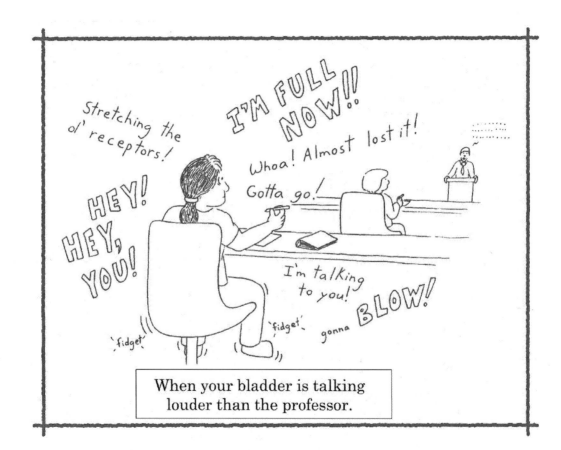

When your bladder is talking louder than the professor.

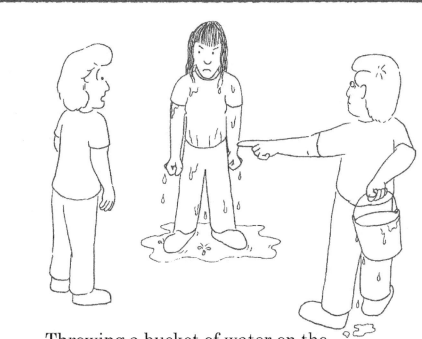

Throwing a bucket of water on the anatomy professor *doesn't* cause her to melt.

You feel like Gilligan in a class full of Professors.

A guinea pig stampede puts you in the hospital.

You find yourself trying to identify muscle layers
in your chicken sandwich.

A classmate says to you, "I can't believe you got this far!
You cost me twenty bucks!"

You're in the middle of a surgery when you forget
the righty-tighty/lefty-loosey rule.

You get kicked by a dead horse.

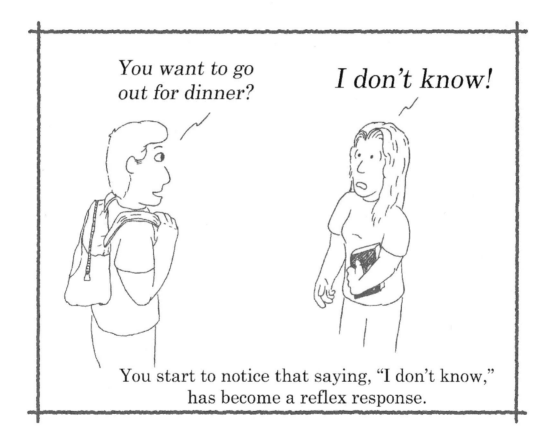

Getting an updated statement in the mail
concerning your financial debt.

Mischievous instructors who come up to you in lab
and say, "Pull my finger."

Crossing your exam threshold and
experiencing anaphylaxis.

You can't remember how that phrase goes –
"Time flies when you're....something, something."

Your levels of dopamine and serotonin
have completely dried up.

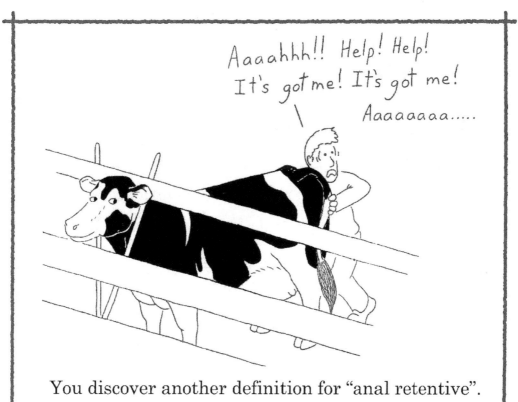

You discover another definition for "anal retentive".

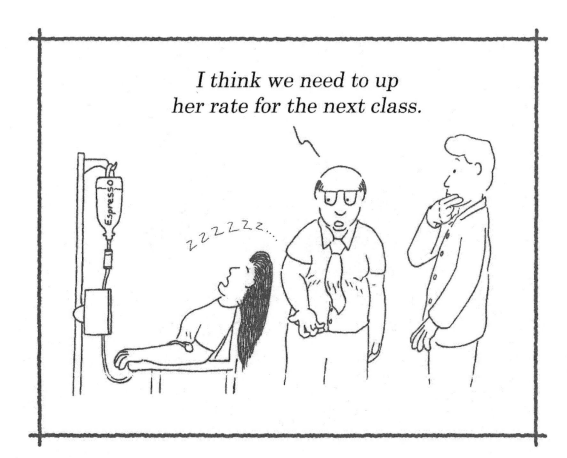

You're told what state and federal laws govern veterinary
medicine at a point when you
really can't turn back.

Fifty-minute class, forty-minute bladder.

You loan your old exams to someone in the year
behind you and they want an explanation
for the grades you received.

You're proud of the 81% you received on a test
and then someone points out that you're
holding your exam upside-down.

You have to look up the word "relax" in the dictionary.

Stop it!
Why are you all staring at me?
I don't have all the answers!

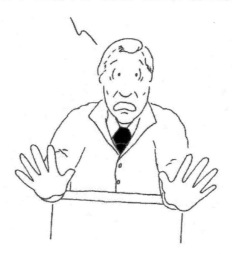

The professor flips out.

You no longer get normal gifts for birthdays and holidays; you get textbooks and veterinary accessories.

You discover sitting in a corn field for prolonged periods of time pretending to be a stalk is quite soothing.

Being accused of cheating on an exam
where you got a "D".

Studying intensely for two weeks before an exam
only to become too ill to take it.

You're always to the left of the bell curve.

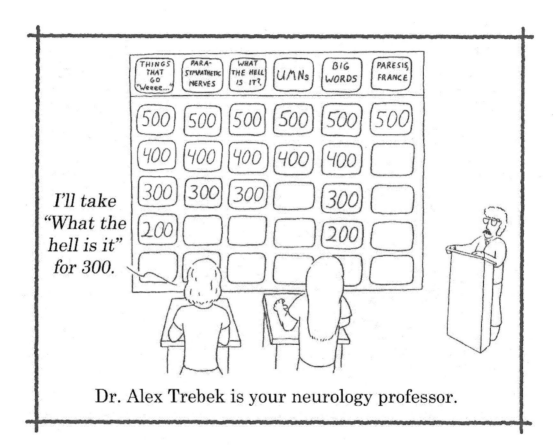

Dr. Alex Trebek is your neurology professor.

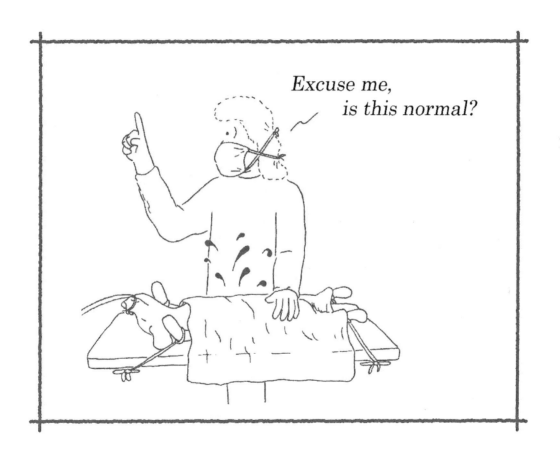

You get to school and find you've studied
for the wrong exam.

Instructors who went into teaching instead
of singing, which they do better.

Research shows that 90% of faculty have
only parasympathetic nerves.

You finally see the "Big Picture" and are blinded.

When you ask a professor how to do better in his class,
his advice is, "You must try harder."

Second year.

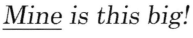

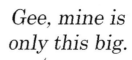

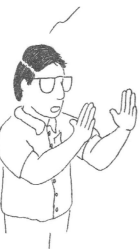

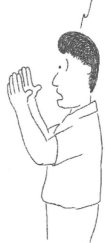

Professors with syllabus envy

Reading all of the suggested references and still
not doing well in the class.

A fellow classmate is taken away in a straight-jacket.

When you ask a serious question, everyone thinks
you're joking, and you never get an answer.

You realize that this program was
completely voluntary.

The emergency loan check you try to cash bounces.

They change the locks on the teaching hospital
and intentionally don't tell you.

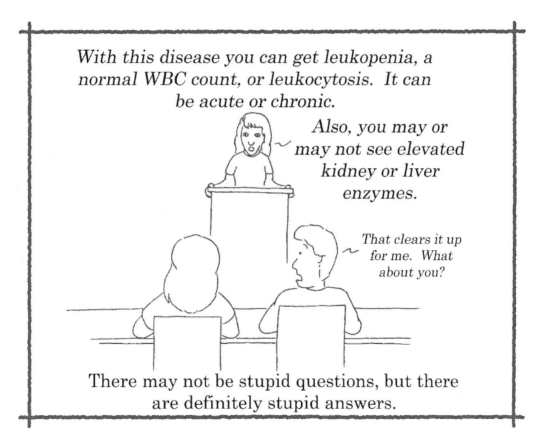

There may not be stupid questions, but there are definitely stupid answers.

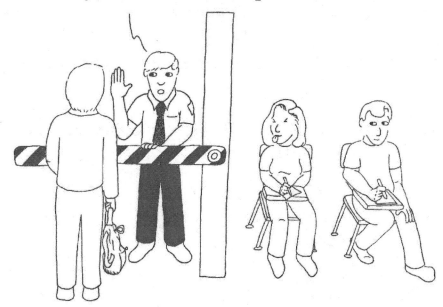

Not being allowed to emigrate to the back row.

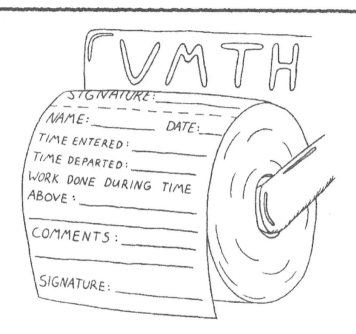

Yet another form

Not only does your school not have a "no bullying" policy,
the professors and clinicians have a strict quota
to meet under their Bullying Protocol.

Third year.

You can't quite get that "laying on of hands" trick down
that the clinicians do at the teaching hospital.

Knowing you'll look back on all of this and not laugh.

Your IRS auditor tells you that he tried to
get into vet school seven times, was never accepted,
and is bitter to this day.

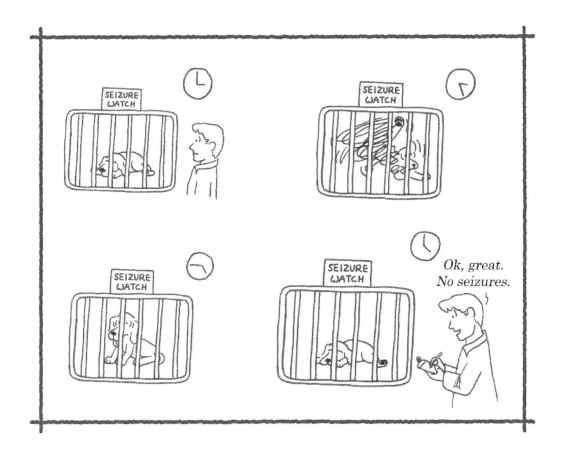

51

A vet student in a previous life

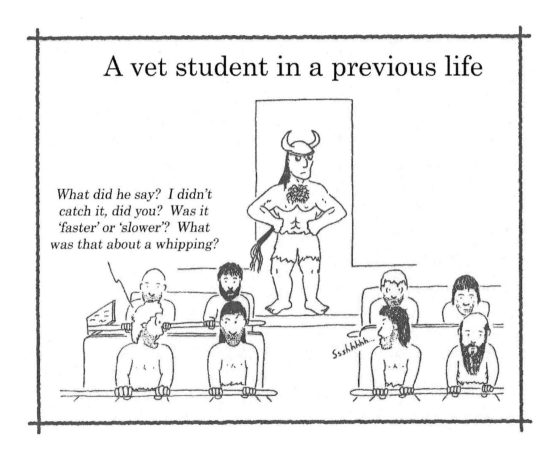

You have to sit at a separate table at family dinners because you "haven't been the same since vet school."

The end of the prepatent period for your unknowingly-acquired Cryptosporidia comes as you sit down for boards.

Medical students on campus "moo" at you.

You find pharmacology makes more sense when read right to left.

People who suggest activities for your "spare" time.

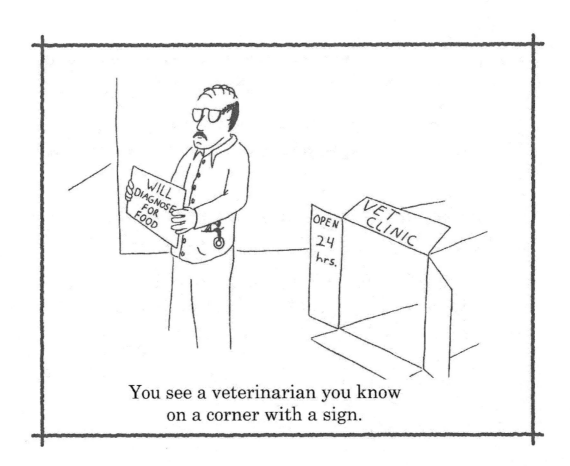

You see a veterinarian you know
on a corner with a sign.

Getting into a fist-fight with a classmate
over who's the most stressed.

You decide it's time to do your laundry when
your clothes refuse to wear you.

Getting the "What's your favorite color" question
in rounds and blowing it.

You keep hearing that the school you attend
is the best in the nation and can't help but wonder, "What's
the criteria?"

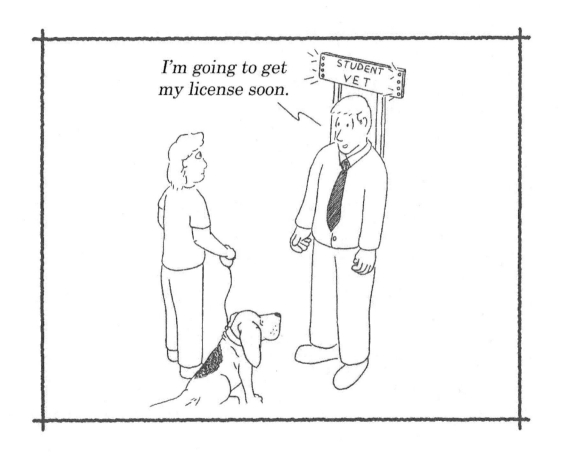

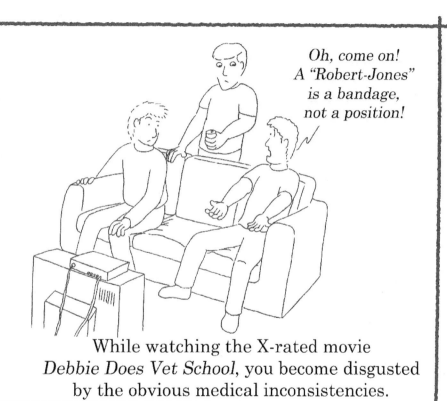

While watching the X-rated movie
Debbie Does Vet School, you become disgusted
by the obvious medical inconsistencies.

Your fortune cookie reads, "What do you think you're doing? Go home! Study!"

The clinician corrects you in front of a client and says that Sneezy, Dopey, Happy, Bashful, Sleepy, Grumpy, and Doc is not a good differential list for PU/PD.

At the scholarship awards ceremony, someone asks, "Why are _you_ here?"

Getting a patient in the hospital with a disease-process you haven't been tested on.

It could happen to anyone!

Mike

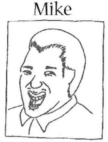

"It's no joking matter. Because of my ignorance, my face is like this permanently."
- Mike

More cases are reported every day!

Flehmen maims!

Don't let this happen to you!

2017 National Flehmen
Poster Child

Doctors are working round-the-clock to develop a preventative vaccine for this plague. Flehmen doesn't kill - oh, no - it is crueler, leaving the victim's maxillary and mandibular labia frozen in a grotesque grimace of a flehmen response.

It's too late for Mike, but who will be next - you?

Formaldehyde doesn't bother you anymore since you haven't really been able to smell anything since first year anatomy.

Sneezing on a blood-agar plate and growing a previously unknown organism.

Hearing about continuing education courses you'll be able to take when you get out of school. yay.

Always being a quarter behind in understanding things.

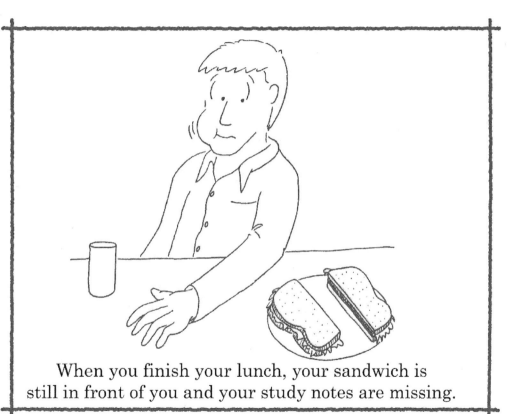

When you finish your lunch, your sandwich is
still in front of you and your study notes are missing.

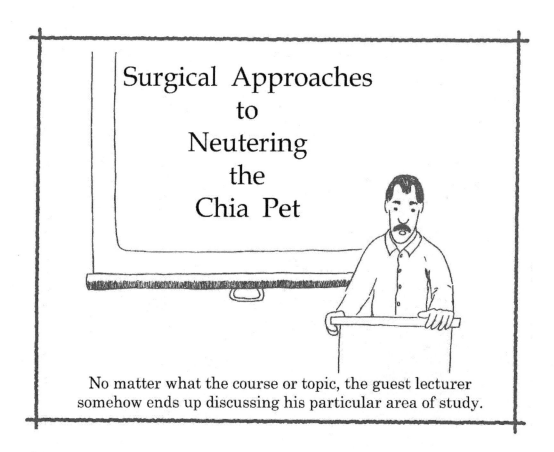

Surgical Approaches
to
Neutering
the
Chia Pet

No matter what the course or topic, the guest lecturer somehow ends up discussing his particular area of study.

The class you're taking is a joke, but you never seem
to get to the punch-line.

After perusing the exam just handed out, you have to
ask the person next to you what class this is.

Being frustrated because you can only do
nine things simultaneously.

Given a choice between paper or plastic,
you can't commit yourself.

45 rpm lectures given at 33$_{1/3}$ rpms or vice-versa.

(ask an older person if you just don't get this reference)

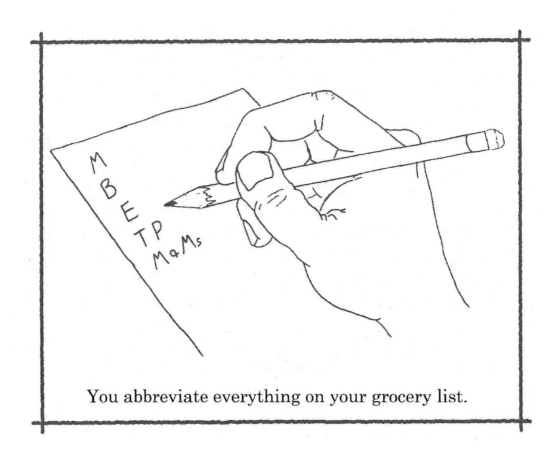

You abbreviate everything on your grocery list.

The Humane Society wants you to be their poster-child to show what can happen when indiscriminate breeding is allowed.

You remember a time when you used to listen to music, not taped-lectures, in the car.

Finding you have a cerebral malabsorption problem.

You've been classified as a type-AAA personality.

People who agree with you when you say, "I just don't think I'm going to make it as a veterinarian."

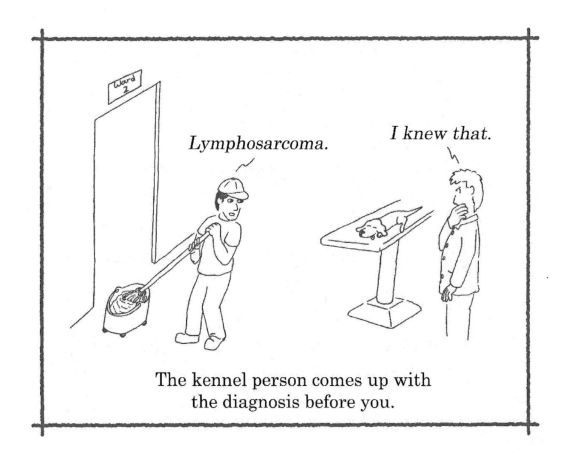

The kennel person comes up with
the diagnosis before you.

Do you ... find yourself with the attention span of a two-year-old?
... find yourself afflicted by malabsorption of information
(ie. mental diarrhea)?
... find yourself having masochistic tendencies?

Well, it's not a tumor! It's Second Year Syndrome (SYS)!*

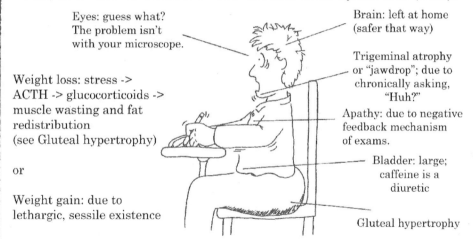

Eyes: guess what? The problem isn't with your microscope.

Brain: left at home (safer that way)

Trigeminal atrophy or "jawdrop"; due to chronically asking, "Huh?"

Weight loss: stress -> ACTH -> glucocorticoids -> muscle wasting and fat redistribution (see Gluteal hypertrophy)

Apathy: due to negative feedback mechanism of exams.

or

Bladder: large; caffeine is a diuretic

Weight gain: due to lethargic, sessile existence

Gluteal hypertrophy

* often goes into remission for a few months, but can recrudesce
as the much more severe Third Year Syndrome (TYS)

Being on the Dean's "other" list.

Being unable to enjoy animals like you used to because you keep seeing them in terms of disease conditions.

During your reproductive ambulatory rotation, you spend fifteen minutes searching for the ovaries before the client walks up to you and asks, "Hey, kid, watch ya' got your arm up that steer's butt for?"

You start to feel that a 400-page syllabus is an acceptable amount of material for one quarter.

Discovering that in live animals, nothing is labeled.

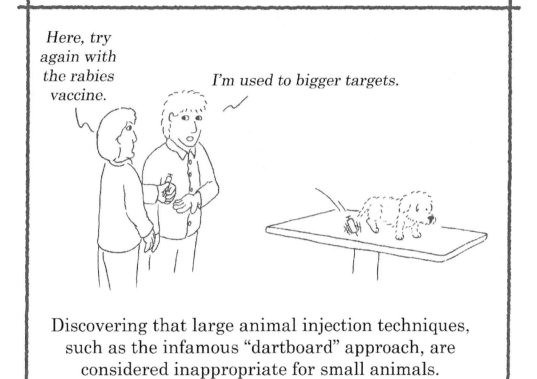

Discovering that large animal injection techniques, such as the infamous "dartboard" approach, are considered inappropriate for small animals.

After asking a professor to review your exam,
you end up with a lower grade.

The only response the administration has to address
grievances is to hand out anti-inflammatories.

Your phone refuses to take any more messages from
"your whiny vet school friends".

Hearing about classmates who "took the weekend off"
and not understanding what that means.

Discovering James Herriot lied.

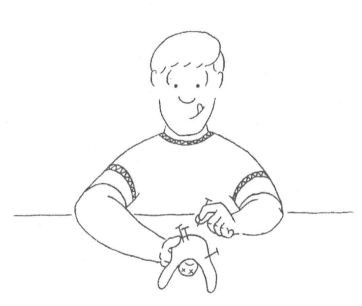

Realizing that you've spent more time making a voodoo doll of the professor than you've spent studying for his exam.

Knowing now in your fourth year why senior students have always looked so much older.

Your horoscope on the Monday of finals week reads: "You feel unprepared for life's challenges.
A good week to avoid testing your abilities.
The letters D and F predominate."

You have to take out an emergency loan to repay your previous emergency loan.

Sitting for two hours at your desk and realizing you haven't turned a page.

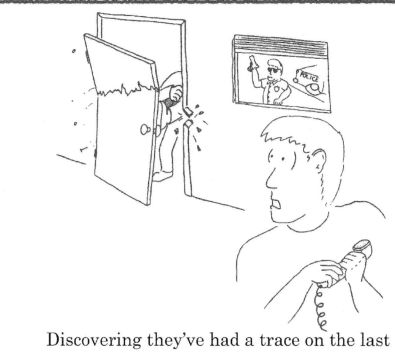

Discovering they've had a trace on the last
five crank calls you made to the professor's house.

You're eligible for a spot on a hemorrhoid commercial
just because you're in vet school.

Extra-curricular activities where you learn more
than you ever have in class.

The future valedictorian of your class is wearing
a t-shirt that reads, "I guess, therefore I am."

The senior student you're assigned to follow and learn from
keeps ditching you in the teaching hospital.

The faculty like you so much they want you around
for another year.

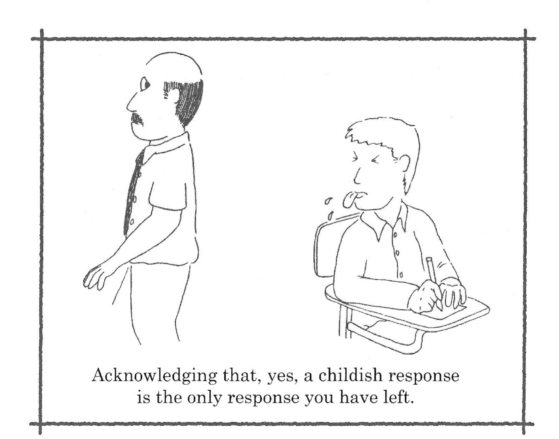

Acknowledging that, yes, a childish response
is the only response you have left.

Having to get an emergency loan to bribe a
professor into raising your grade.

Getting lost and accidentally stumbling across
the teaching hospital's torture room.

Hypoglycemia becomes a way of life.

The "spring forward, fall back" rule for time-change also
applies to your grades.

Pulling a muscle when lifting your copy of Ettinger.

You see your picture on the back of a milk carton.

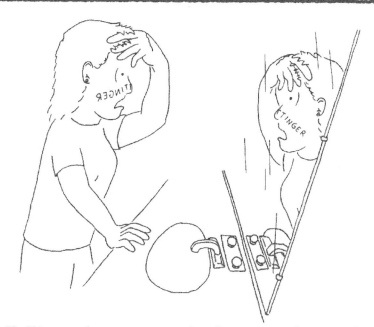

Falling asleep on your book causes the word
"Ettinger" to be imprinted permanently on your face.

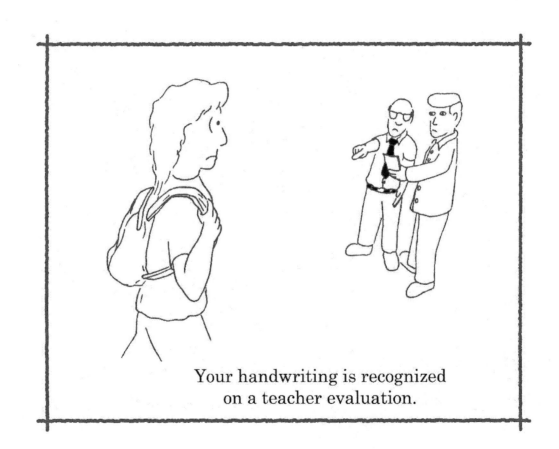

Your handwriting is recognized
on a teacher evaluation.

First through third year students
being referred to as "whelps".

Being told what stress-reduction books you can read when
you have no time to read them.

You wonder why, if evaluations are considered and
responded to, there are still so many poor instructors.

Given a choice between vet school and crucifixion, you're
undecided.

The lecturer doesn't know the answer to
25-down either.

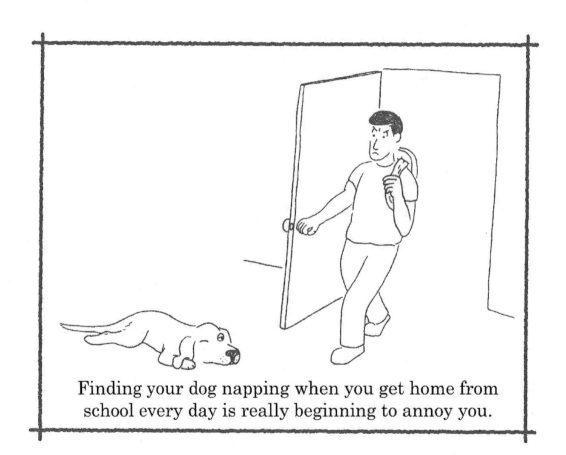

Finding your dog napping when you get home from school every day is really beginning to annoy you.

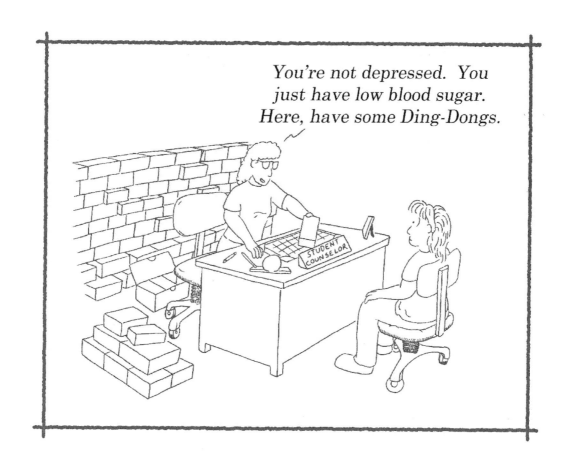

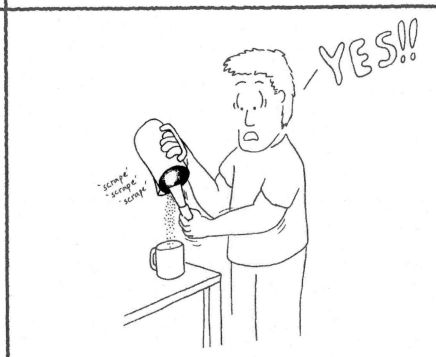

You find the three-day-old coffee acceptable during finals.

You have a continuing nightmare involving the rubral spinal tract and a wombat with an Australian accent.

A 7.0 unit class with only one test – the final.

After seeing the amount of paperwork that
is done at the teaching hospital,
you know exactly where the rain forests are going.

Watching "Lifestyles of the Rich and Famous" and noting
there's not a veterinarian among them.

The vending machine only contains
non-caffeinated, diet drinks.

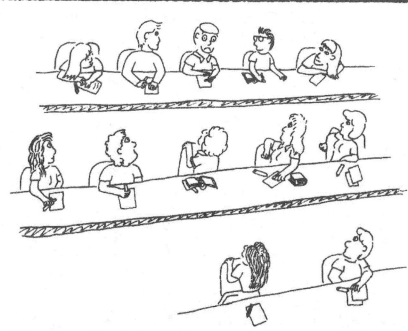

Everyone turns to look at you when you ask
your first question in class in three years.

A homeless person looks at you, looks towards the sky, and
mutters, "There, but for the grace of God, go I."

You are told that, no, hematuria is not a star
in the Orion Nebula.

You go to the financial aid office
and they ask you for a loan.

You have to ask someone what "social life" means.

Being able to diagnose yourself as having
Cushing's disease.

And I would also like to thank
the creators of caffeine
for making all of this possible.

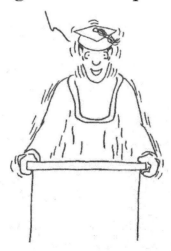

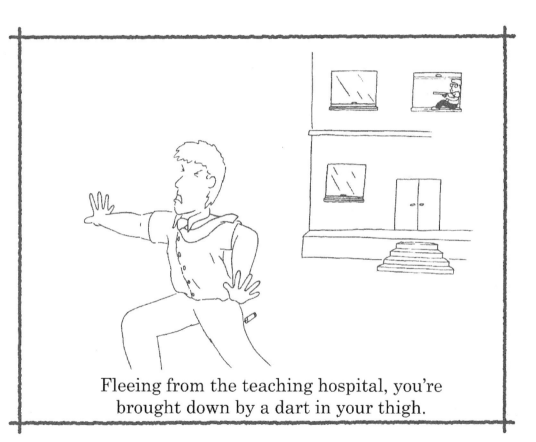

Fleeing from the teaching hospital, you're brought down by a dart in your thigh.

Dr._____(fill in name of most stressful professor)

Finding that there might be a better way to choose
medications for patients than "one-potato, two-potato".

Someone who says, "Aren't you too young
to be a veterinarian?"

Getting exams returned in your third year
from classes you took in your second year.

You find yourself highlighting pertinent points
in newspaper articles.

No one takes you seriously any more.

Fourth year.

You get to Day Twenty in the required computer
case-simulation and discover......there's more.

Someone who says, "Aren't you too old
to be a veterinary student?"

Getting an endocrine question wrong and having to do ten
"Our Professors" and five "Hail Deans" as penance.

Classes that continue into a second quarter.

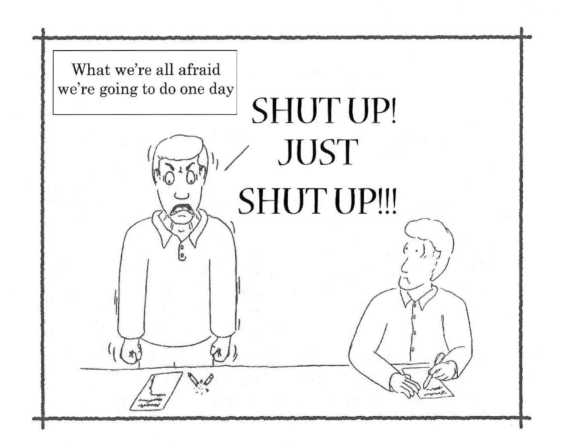

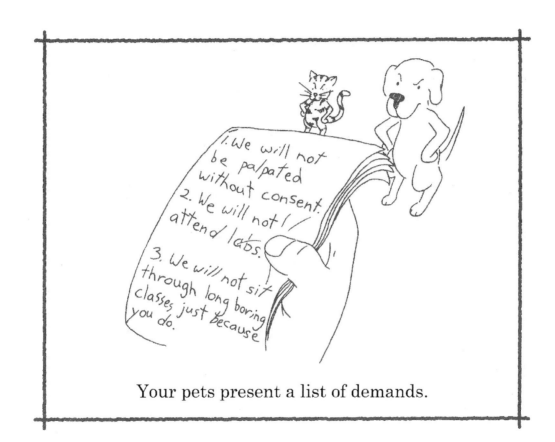

Your pets present a list of demands.

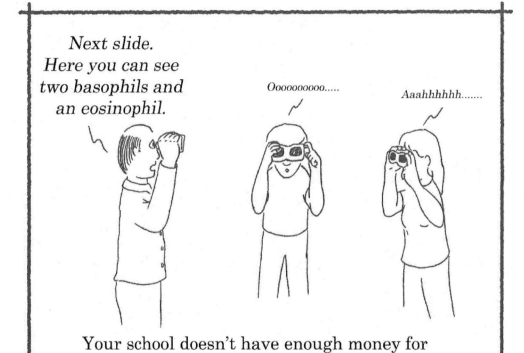

Your school doesn't have enough money for microscopes so it uses ViewMasters.

Suffering from Vitamin D deficiency
since you never see the sun.

Fifth year.

Constantly hearing about human diseases in class.

The small animal clinic at the teaching hospital: where
they worry more about how you look
than what you learn.

Labs that are really three-hour lectures.

You get the sample question wrong.

Don't worry. There are only
forty of us in the herd.

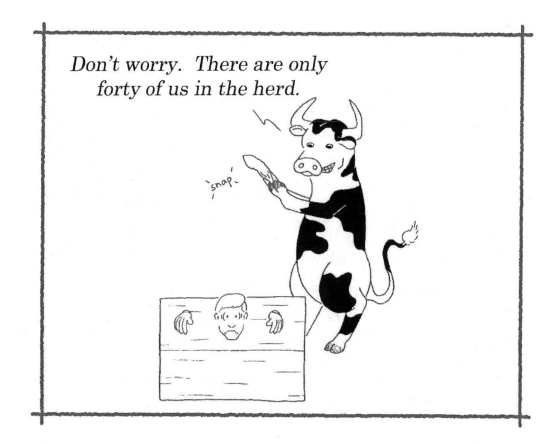

The only answers you get right on the
National Boards are the ones they throw out.

The sound of your stomach mucosa sloughing
is disturbing the other test-takers
and you are asked to leave.

During finals you decide to forego the bathroom visit when
you hear about the body cavity search.

You find small suspicious-looking electrodes
hooked to your metal chair.

You no longer have deep-pain sensation.

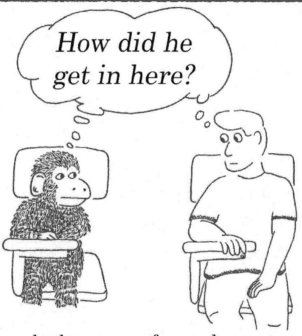

You wonder how some of your classmates
could possibly have been accepted.

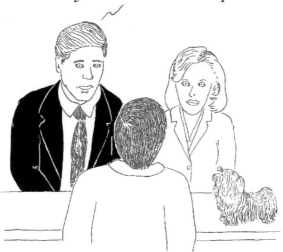

We have reason to believe that the only explanation for Lhasa Apsos is that they're from another planet.

Your next case is straight from _The X-Files_.

Three months of intense, six-hour-per-day studying for the State and National Boards was ill-used.

Having just put in the last suture, thus completing your first live surgery, you can only account for three out of four hemostats.

A class is so boring that you form a lick granuloma on your forearm.

They discover the notes you sent out in hopes of rescue.

You spend $200 on a book only to find out that a new edition is coming out next month.

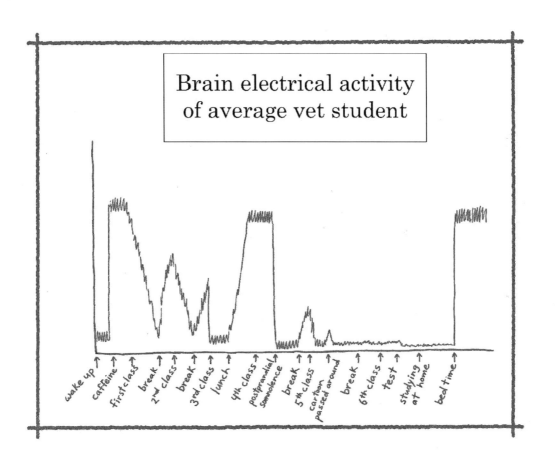

99

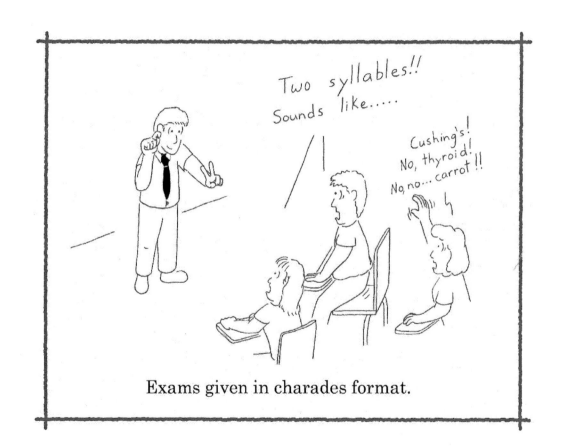

Exams given in charades format.

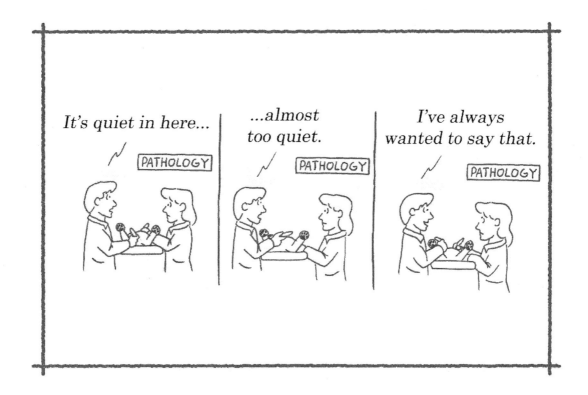

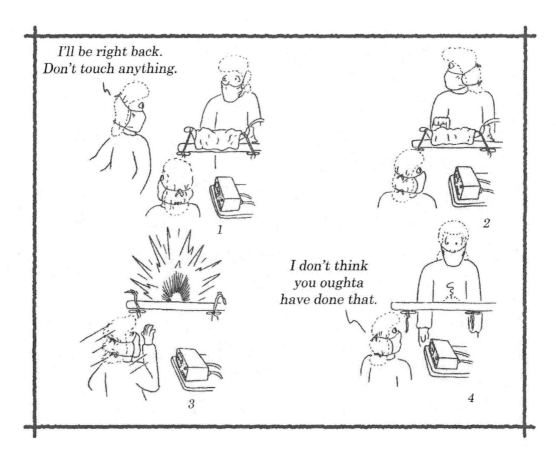

You have the distinct feeling that your cat is trying to tell you something when he buries your notes in the litter box.

When you have to see the Dean about your grades, you notice he has a well-worn copy of *Mein Kampf* on his bookshelf.

Because of the diarrhea you had during the gastrointestinal class, and because of the PU/PD you experienced during renal, and also because of the nervous tic you developed during neurology, you decide to avoid the abnormal reproduction laboratory.

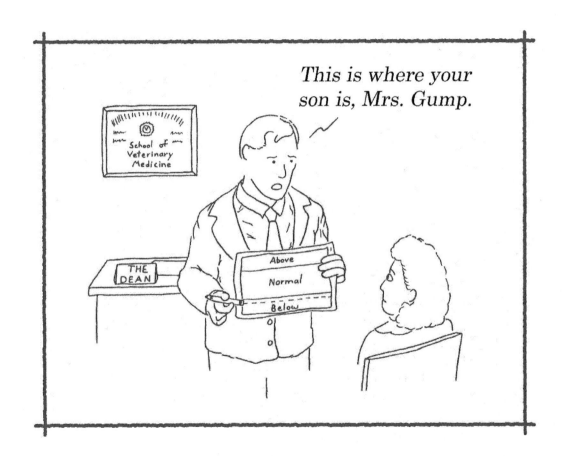

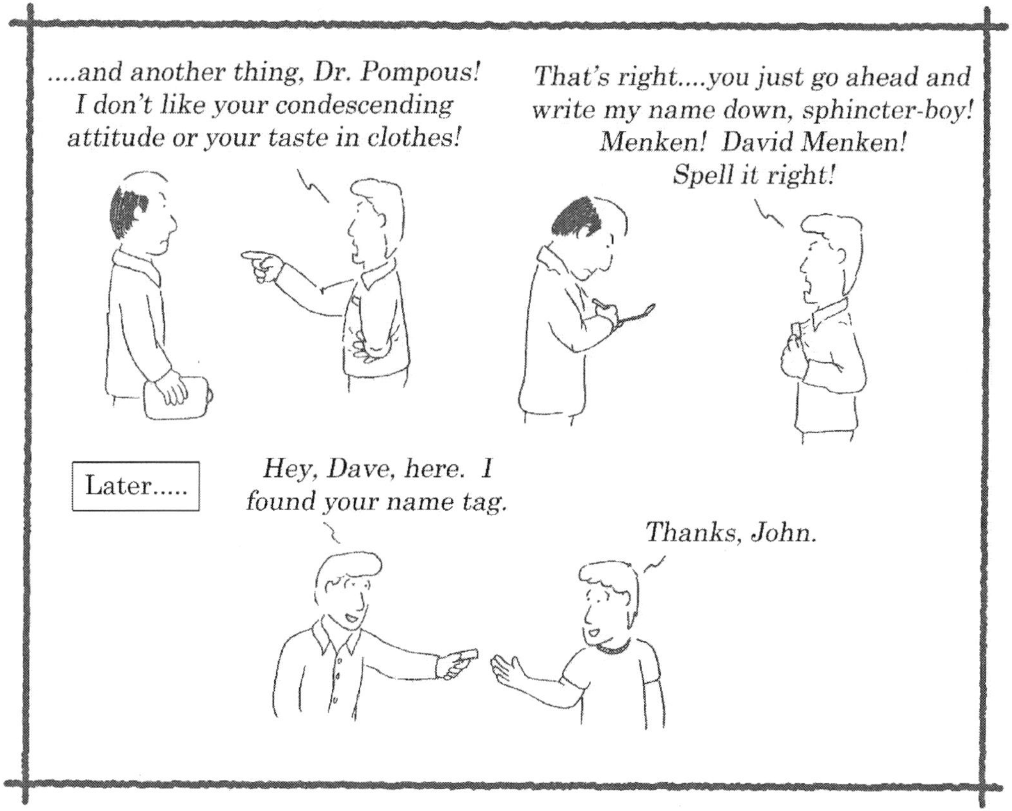
....and another thing, Dr. Pompous! I don't like your condescending attitude or your taste in clothes!
That's right....you just go ahead and write my name down, sphincter-boy! Menken! David Menken! Spell it right!
Later.....
Hey, Dave, here. I found your name tag.
Thanks, John.

You're told "Happiness is a choice", however
your school has chosen for you otherwise.

Your personal physician, who owns an eight-bedroom home
on 100 acres of land and drives a Porsche to work, tells you,
"I started out in vet school, but I dropped out and went to
medical school instead."

You are in the latest JAVMA *What's Your Diagnosis* article
as the patient.

You find out that your pre-veterinary advisor
didn't even have a DVM.

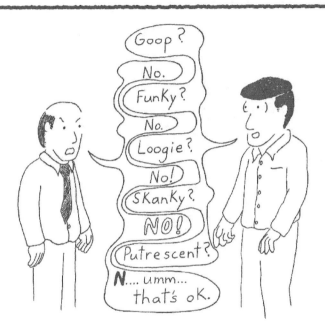

You are asked to please stop using terms such as "oogie", "goober", "grody", and "yucky".

Clinicians that tell you in your fourth year,
"Of course, you won't have the diagnostic capabilities
in private practice that we have here."

Being referred to as "piñata-boy" during rounds.

While you are signing the Student Oath at the end of the
test to affirm that you didn't cheat,
the person next to you whispers,
"Thanks for letting me see your answers."

Realizing that the last time you got a 100
was on a 200-point test.

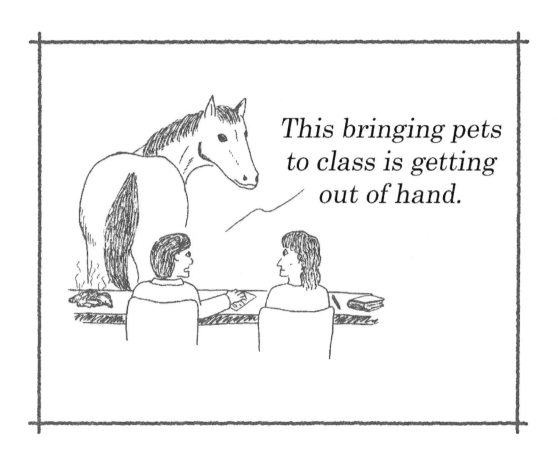

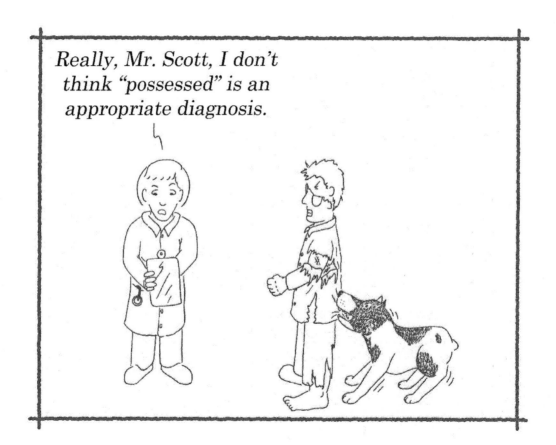

Suddenly realizing that class has been over for forty minutes and you're alone in the room.

Professor who, when leaving class, uses a fake Austrian accent to say, "I'll be back."

Your psychiatrist has heard just about enough out of you!

A 600 page "syllabus".

During your first spay they play the theme to *Mission Impossible*.

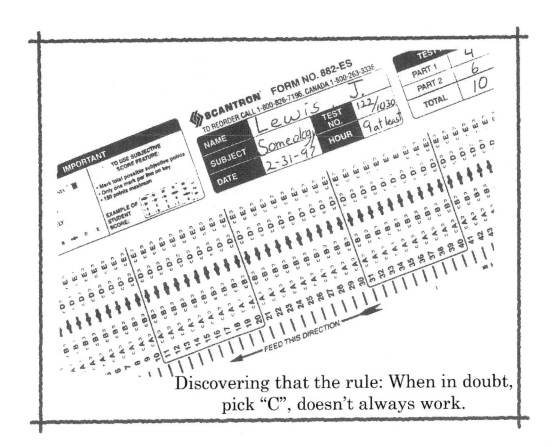

Discovering that the rule: When in doubt,
pick "C", doesn't always work.

They forget to call your name at graduation.

Fluoxetine is your school's drug of choice.

Bringing a Ouija board into clinic rounds
is starting to seem like a good idea.

Your dog chews up your animal behavior textbook.

After complaining about the abusive way students are
treated, the administration responds blandly,
"You aren't covered under the Animal Welfare Act."

A contact lens falls into your surgery site.

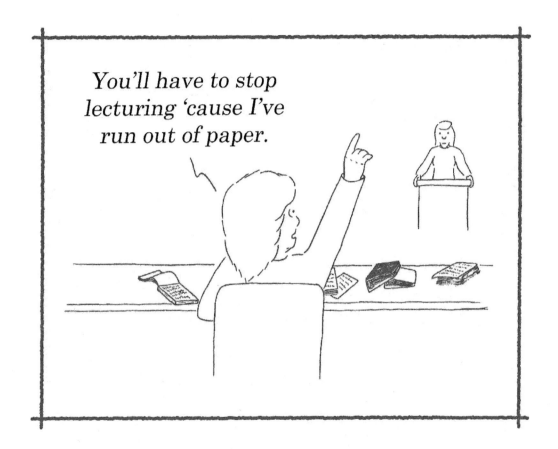

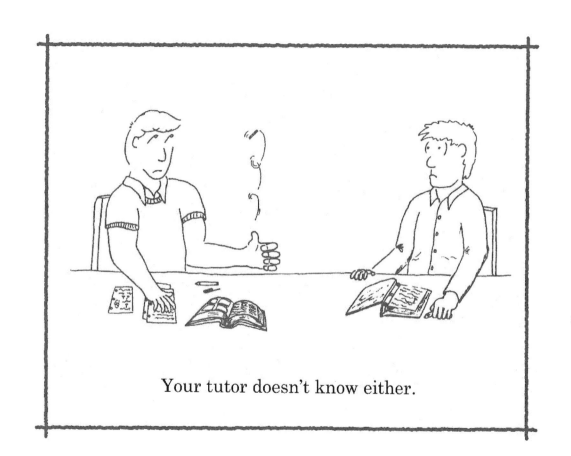

Your tutor doesn't know either.

Having to explain how the endoscope
got stuck up your nose.

You're always picked to be the "catcher"
when they electro-ejaculate the bull.

You've applied to the same school so many times you're on
a first-name basis with the board members.

In your final year of vet school, your school
loses its accreditation.

Having to learn about animal species that you know you
will never treat once you become a veterinarian.

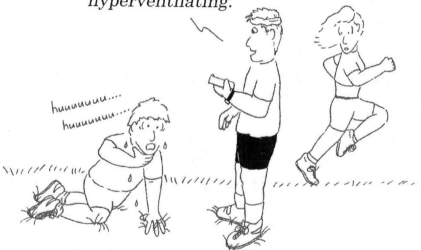

Classmates who feel obligated to
relate everything to medicine.

You find out that when you took the National Boards, CCT, and State Boards, all you passed was gas.

You overhear a classmate refer to student loans as "paying for your mistake".

You discover that exercise reduces your stress level, but you're spending sixteen hours a day in the gym.

You try and try, but in reproductive surgery you're only able to do a D-section.

A clinician rubs your nose in the surgery site saying, "Bad. That was bad, baaaaddd….."

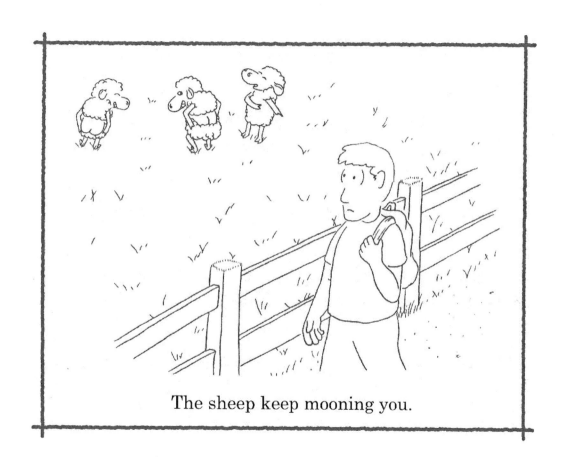

The sheep keep mooning you.

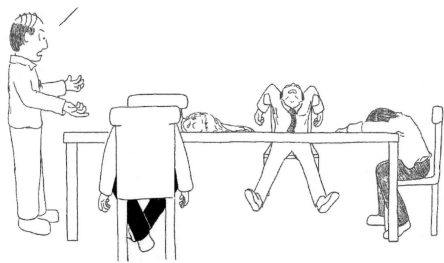

Oh, c'mon......you can't <u>all</u> be dead!

To avoid answering questions in rounds,
you pretend to be dead.

Upon entering the teaching hospital, you hear
a threatening, ghostly voice hissing, "Get out......"

You recall laughing at veterinarians who tried to warn you
away from vet school. Oh, how you laughed.

Optional classes that you skip and later
you hear were damn useful.

Sex is a vague and distant memory.

You have to look up what the word "sex" means.

Your limbic system is really taking a beating.

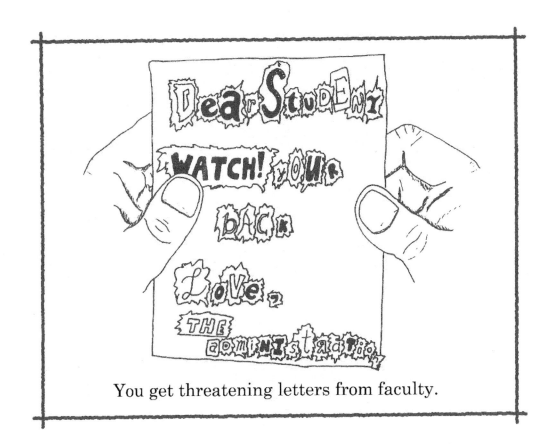

You get threatening letters from faculty.

Because there is no "alternatives" program,
you have to sacrifice you own life for vet school.

You're the only one who didn't know that the take-home
clinical questions were based on actual teaching hospital
cases and all the answers could be called up on the hospital
computers.

Professors who should start all of their lectures with,
"Once upon a time....",
because they invariably put you to sleep.

Your GI professor seems to be pulling
questions out of his ass.

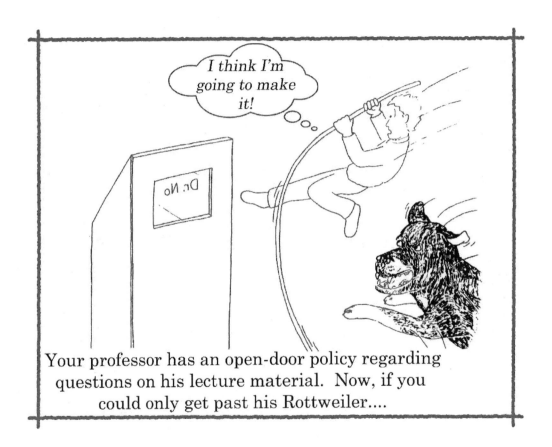

Your professor has an open-door policy regarding questions on his lecture material. Now, if you could only get past his Rottweiler....

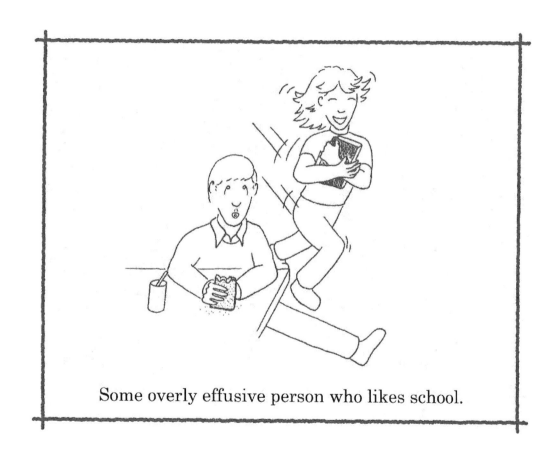

Some overly effusive person who likes school.

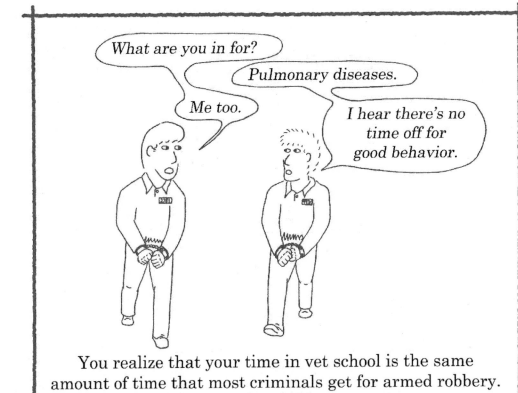

You realize that your time in vet school is the same amount of time that most criminals get for armed robbery.

While you are mopping up after your patient, a clinician walks by and says, "It's good to work on your secondary skills in case your primary ones don't work out."

You've started to notice more uses for the F-word since you've been in school.

You keep writing your parents about how hard vet school is and the letters keep coming back marked "Return to Sender".

People ask you veterinary information relating to their pets but don't believe what you tell them.

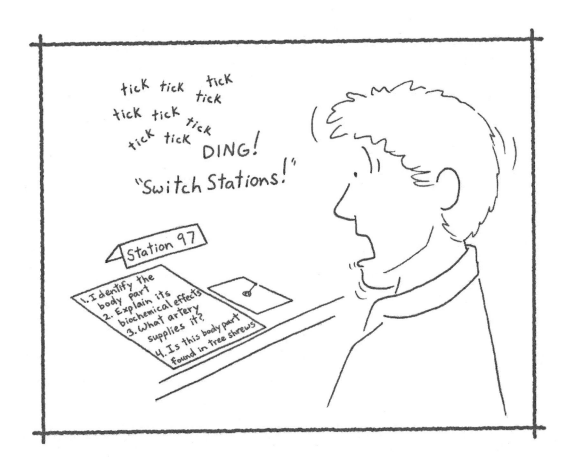

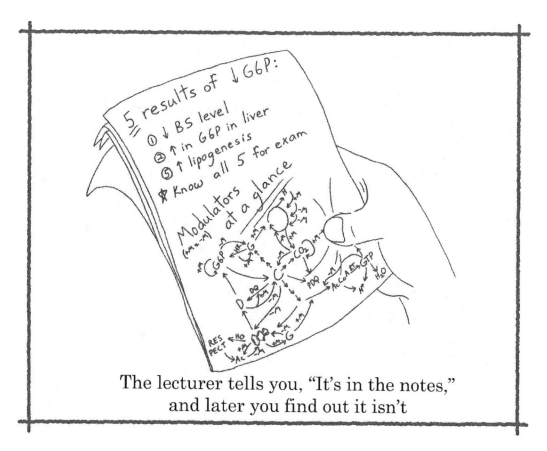

The lecturer tells you, "It's in the notes,"
and later you find out it isn't

After stopping to consider all the animals you've stuck with
sharp needles since you started on this educational path,
you begin to worry that their descendants
are going to one day seek revenge.

You, your classmate, and the ultrasound machine
are caught in an embarrassing menage a trois.

You're informed that "purpleocyte", "thingamaphage", and
"guessophil" are not recognized hematology terms.

You call up random people and ask if you can
borrow their dog, just for a few minutes.

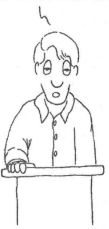

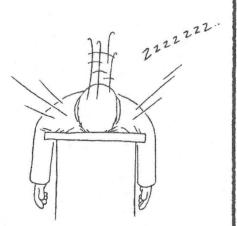

The lecturer is so boring he puts himself to sleep.

You scream "I've got a knife!"
at people who try to sell you things.

You scream "I've got a knife!"
at people during the family reunion.

You like cats. Especially with mayo.

You start listing things that stress you out.

You start scheduling your vacations
in fifty-minute blocks of time.

Your grades spell out Elmer's last name.

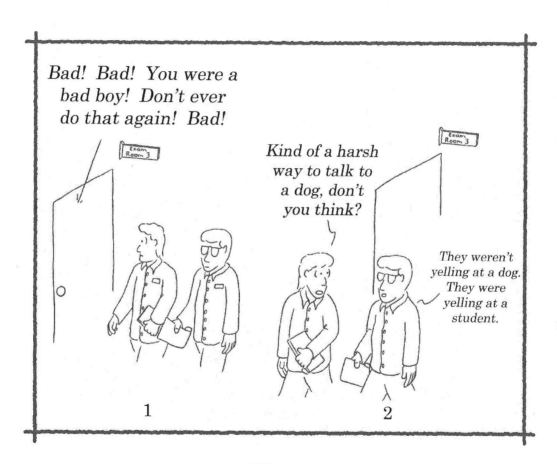

133

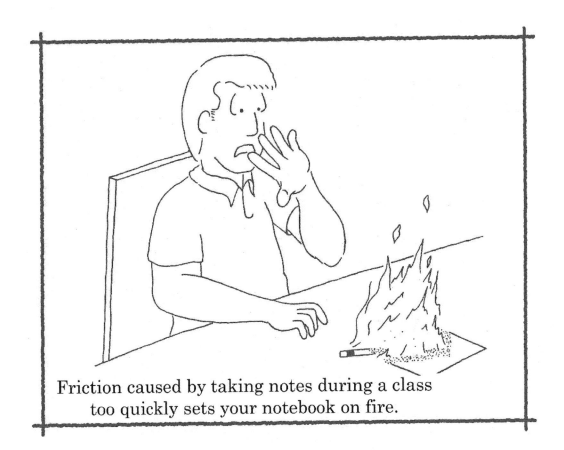

Friction caused by taking notes during a class
too quickly sets your notebook on fire.

Classmates who say, "When I see you, I think, well, I really don't have it that bad."

You argue with a classmate about which is better — to be eaten by a koala bear or to be loved by an infectious disease. And you spend hours referencing information to back-up your claim.

The only response you can come up with on an exam is, "This page intentionally left blank".

You start to palpate the abdomen of the client's male dog and the client exclaims in an outraged voice, "What do you think you are doing?!"

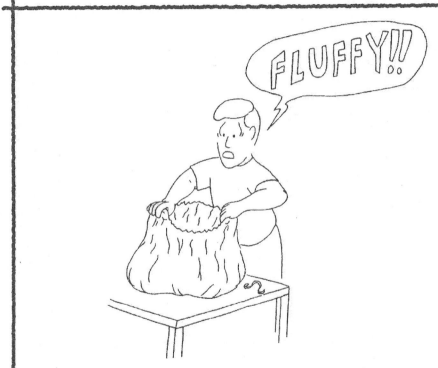

Your pathology specimen looks familiar.

The professor is getting angry with the victory dance you do after each question you answer correctly.

You find out that you and four other classmates are being traded to another vet school for better students.

The repeated thudding of your head on the desk wakes up your classmates.

You start to notice a trend. You came from a dysfunctional family and now you're entering a dysfunctional profession. Hmmmmm........

You discover you're in an educational LD50 study.

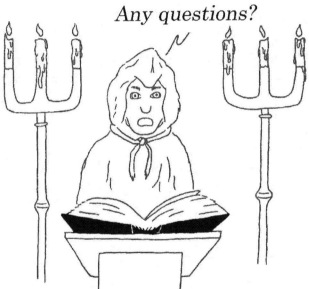

Classes given in the ancient language of Acronymia.

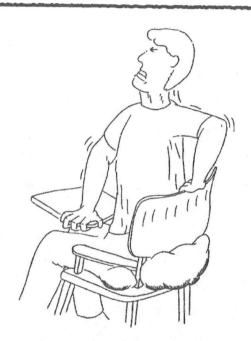

Upon trying to stand up after four hours of lectures, you find your butt is wedged in the chair due to venous pooling.

You become impatient at the amount of time
your microwave popcorn takes.

You're diagnosed with a learning disability late in your
fourth year, and while that certainly explains a lot, it's not
very useful information at this point.

All of your classmates are wearing the same shirt
that reads, "We're With Stupid".

Having to take ever-increasing doses of motion-sickness
medicine to get through all of the cytology slides.

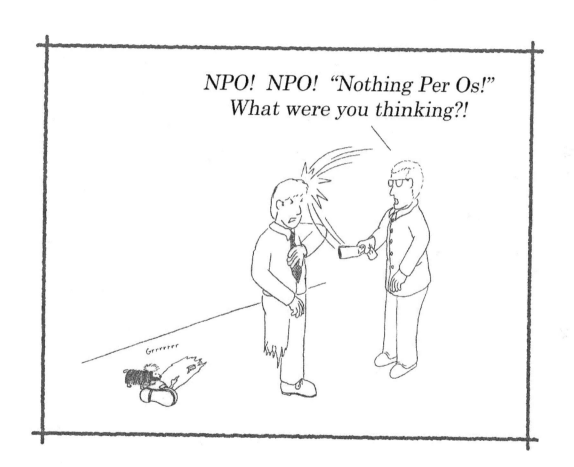

Getting withdrawal symptoms whenever you haven't
sat in class or touched a textbook for too long.

The Exam Gods are displeased.

Euthanasia is not an option.

You no longer have a diurnal rhythm.

A classmate, who scored higher than you, says,
"Wow, the only time I studied for this
was like an hour before the test! Crazy, right?"

Some of your classmates have tan lines.

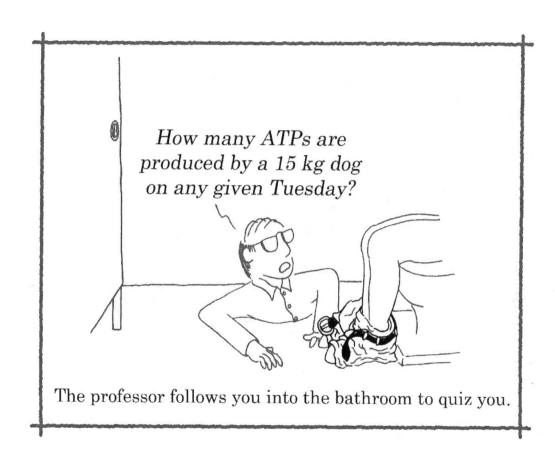

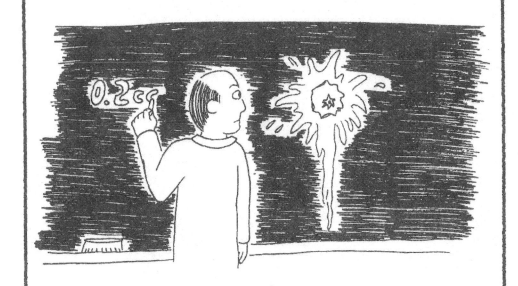

You miss the professor with thrown rotten fruit.

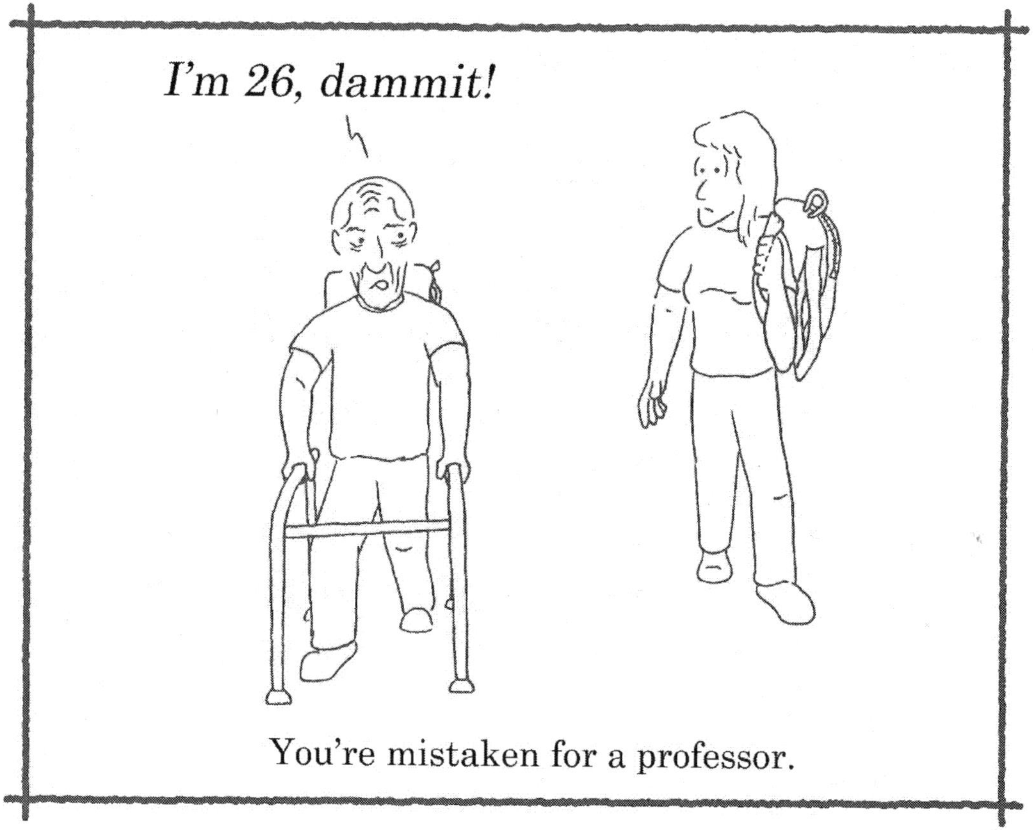

You're mistaken for a professor.

Every time a resident or clinician approaches,
you urinate submissively.

Finding more and quicker ways to spend your money.

Getting kicked by a sheep, a cow, a horse,
and a clinician all in the same day.

You keep trying to convince yourself that,
even though most of your classmates have only three years
of undergrad school, you're really glad
you got your B.S. degree. No, really.

Classmates who are ethically-challenged.

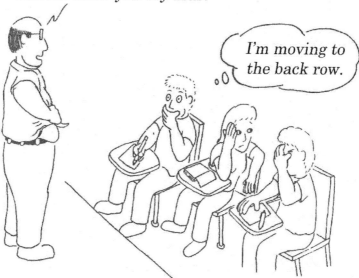

You learn more about your physiology professor's personal biology than you ever wanted to know.

Submitted for your approval.
A 200 question, multiple choice
test, with 26 choices per question,
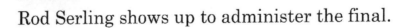 *and more than one choice*
is correct......

Rod Serling shows up to administer the final.

Your nocturnal studying behavior is interfering with your pets' sleep and they politely ask you to STOP IT!

The professor doesn't cast a reflection in the mirror.

You find it to be an unusual social quirk that your classmates can be just dead-wrong about something and the clinicians and residents will admire their effort. Yet those same people will chastise and berate you if you say, "I don't know, but I'll find out."

The only internship you're offered is at Wossamotta University.

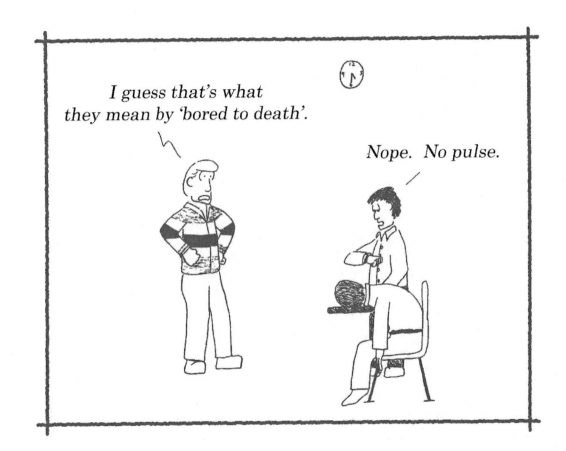

You develop a contact allergy
to your dermatology notes.

The vet school's immune system has
identified you as a foreign protein.

You forget the combination to your school locker.

Sweat in your eyes during surgery.

Reviewing your current student loan status, the loan officer
exclaims, "Wow! That's a lot of zeroes!"

You get 20 points off on a 10 point question.

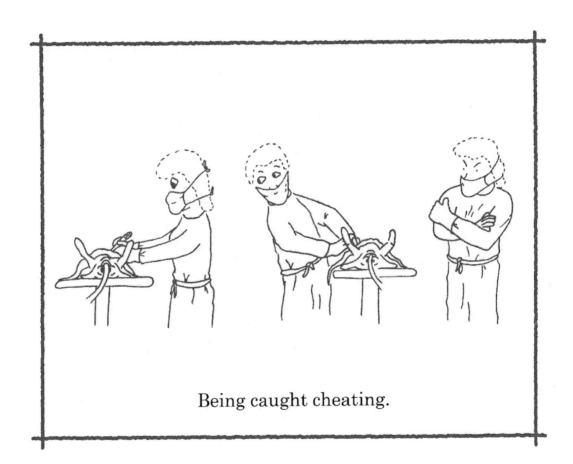

Being caught cheating.

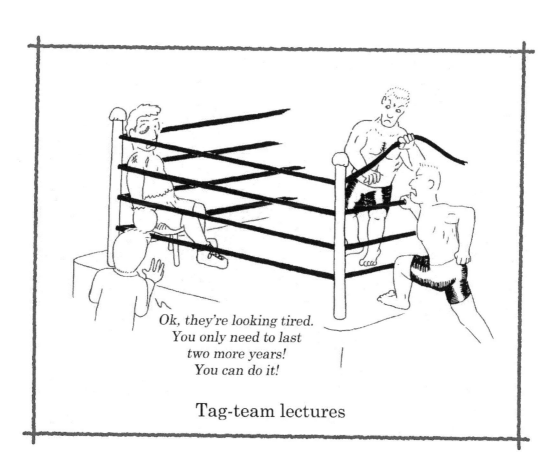

Tag-team lectures

While reading over your notes, you can't remember if the professor said to be able to "recognize but not memorize" or "memorize but not recognize"
the material.

When referencing something from a two-volume text, you always, *always*, **always** have the wrong volume
in your hand first.

After seeing the movie *Outbreak*, about a zoonotic disease epidemic, you realize that there was not one single veterinarian in the whole film.

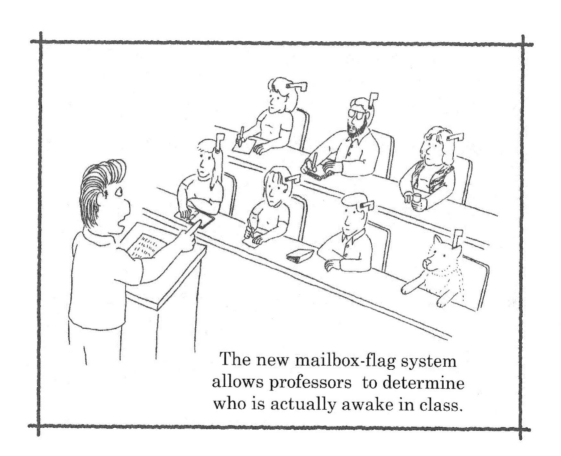

The new mailbox-flag system allows professors to determine who is actually awake in class.

Unfortunately, after the cannabis-effect wears off, endocrinology doesn't make sense any more.

The professor uses the abbreviation "B.Y.O. 'KY'" when discussing the upcoming exam.

Being able to relate to the scarecrow from *The Wizard of Oz*.

Starting the countdown until graduation with Day Five-Hundred and Thirteen.

The ambulatory resident leaves you stranded in "Deliverance"-country.

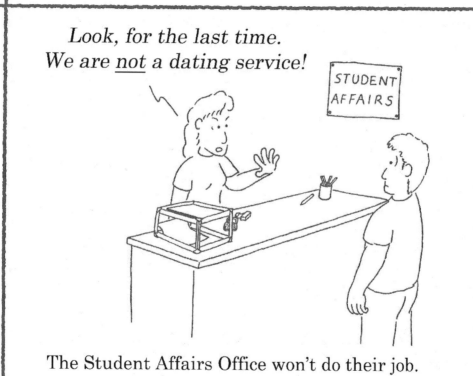

The Student Affairs Office won't do their job.

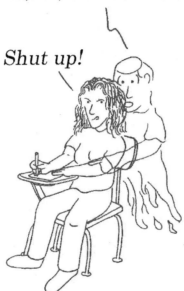

The ghost of a previous student keeps
whispering wrong answers to you during the exam.

You realize that having pathology lectures right before lunch no longer kills your appetite.

After much debate and research, your study group decides that an interrupted-cruciate pattern is most appropriate for sewing a button back on your shirt.

You find it necessary to scrub up to your elbows before using the toilet.

Your classmate slaps your face when you ask, "Have you ever tried a continuous horizontal mattress pattern?"

Graduating in the top 98% of your class.

Realizing at 3 A.M. on the Sunday before finals week that you can make a really cool fort out of all your books.

After a pathology wet-lab focusing on thoracic abnormalities, you find yourself craving barbecued ribs.

Noticing that in the Milton Bradley game *Life*, there's no career option for being a veterinarian.

The professor explains that while, yes, your answer was correct, you didn't say, "Simon Says".

Your significant other keeps asking, "Why do you have to study so much?"

Because of the amount of time spent in classes, your child is raised by a pack of wolves.

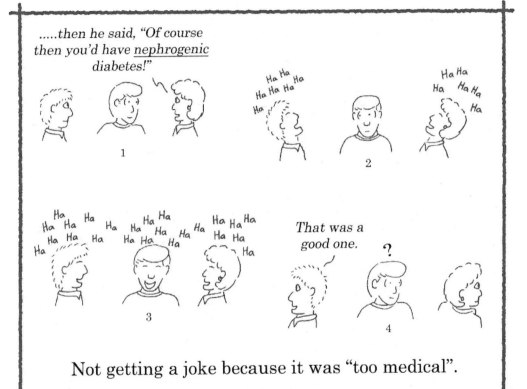

Not getting a joke because it was "too medical".

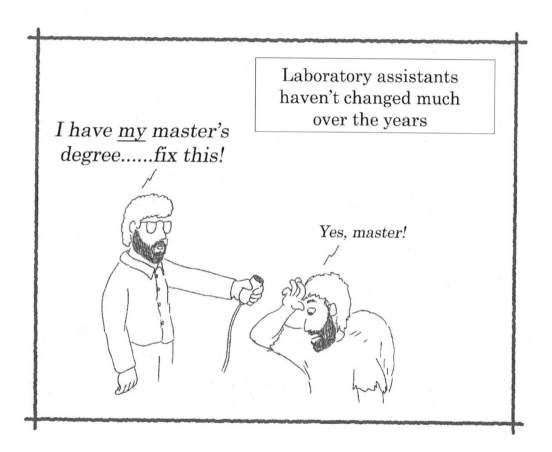

163

Your date reminds you that maggots are not an appropriate topic of conversation in a public restaurant.

You see recurring TV shows about lawyers, doctors, police officers, and lifeguards (for God's sake), but the only veterinary show is, again, PBS's James Herriot.

Having to take classes in vet school that you have already taken since, oddly enough, they were prerequisites for getting into vet school.

You're asked to remove your reclining chair from the classroom.

"Guessing with confidence" isn't working.

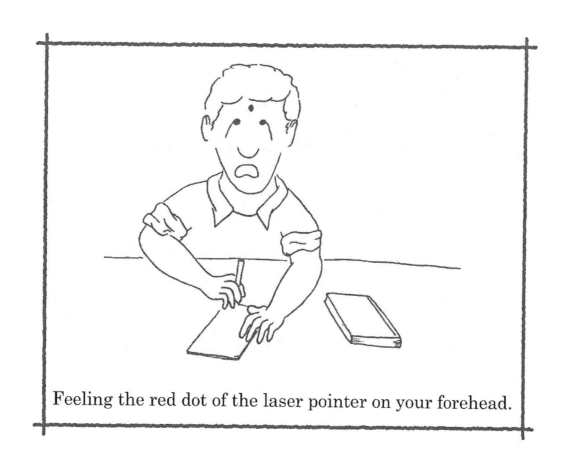

Feeling the red dot of the laser pointer on your forehead.

The professor's shadow keeps blocking the
view of the overhead projector.

Your classmates find you head-pressing
in a corner of the lecture hall.

When there are fourteen differentials,
you're always called on to list the fourteenth.

You find out the hard way that the
"optional" cardiology review wasn't.

Diversity workshops are considered
more essential than anatomy reviews.

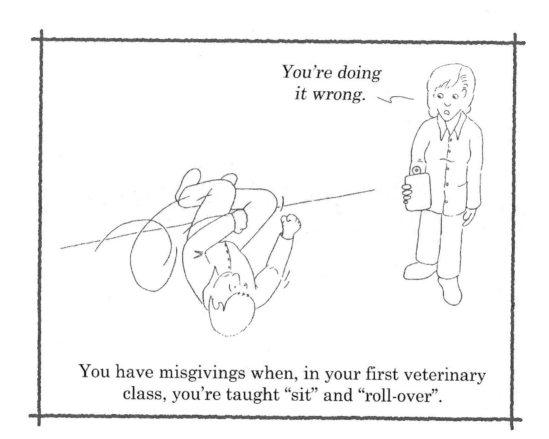

You have misgivings when, in your first veterinary class, you're taught "sit" and "roll-over".

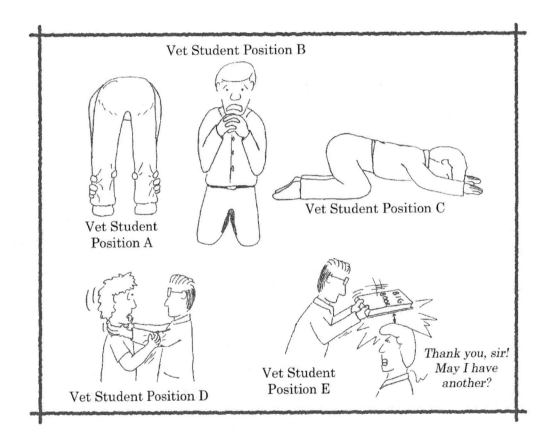

Vet Student Position B

Vet Student Position A

Vet Student Position C

Vet Student Position D

Vet Student Position E

Thank you, sir! May I have another?

You make it across the empty compound and past
the tower guards, but are inescapably
caught in the barbed wire.

The only latex product you've had time to use
are your surgical gloves.

Knowing you've never seen a practicing veterinarian
scrambling to determine the Ideal Alveolar Gas Equation.

You have to take classes with medical students,
but they get graded pass/fail.

The school's motto is "No Pain, No Gain".

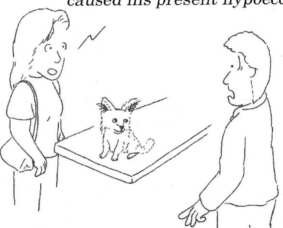

He underwent litholapaxy, but had a recidivation of his elastorrhexis resulting in the need for a transureteroureterostomy which caused his present hypoeccrisia.

A client uses bigger words than you.

You have a house-mate with a high school diploma
who works out of the living room and
makes more than you ever will.

On your first day of rotation, the clinician wanders off and
leaves you to justify his treatment
of a long-term and expensive case to the client.

Trying to explain that, yes, you're a vet student and you
really enjoy animals, but you can't squeeze "just one more"
cat into your household menagerie.

The thousand-and-somethingth person asks,
"So, big or little animals?"

Stomach as balloon,
Twisting, twisting, round and round,
Decompress and soon

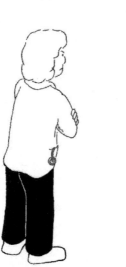
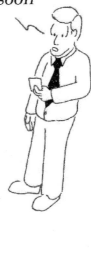

The Emergency Medicine clinician
wants all of your answers in haiku.

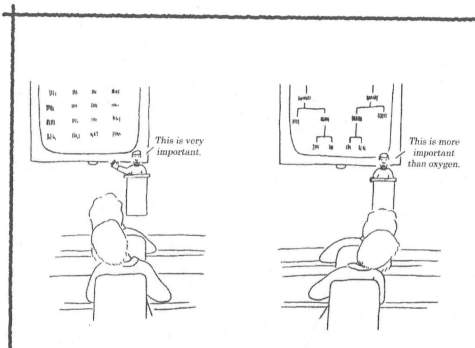

The person in front of you always moves in the same direction when you are trying to see the screen.

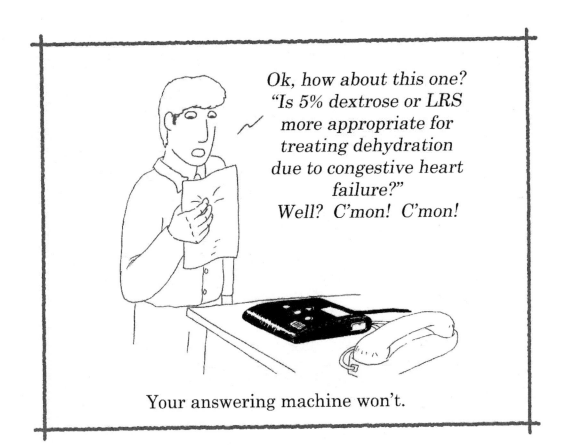

Doing a great work-up and therapy on a patient who dies of natural causes immediately upon leaving the hospital.

Being able to read the lecture syllabus faster than the lecturer can read the syllabus aloud in class.

Being introduced to a new faculty member who says, "Oh, yes, I've heard of *you*."

Dr. Kevorkian is in charge of the school's Human-Animal Bond program.

Reading the insurance liability claims Against Drs. X, Y, and Z.

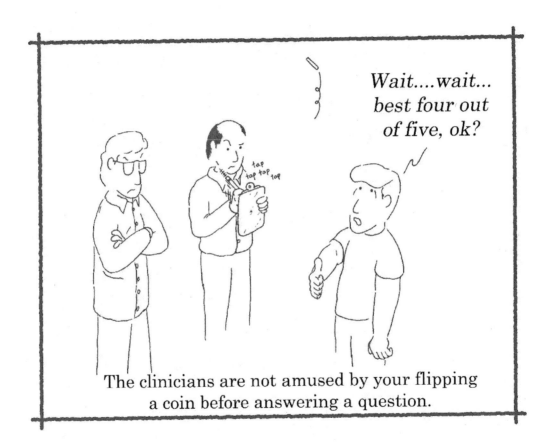

The clinicians are not amused by your flipping
a coin before answering a question.

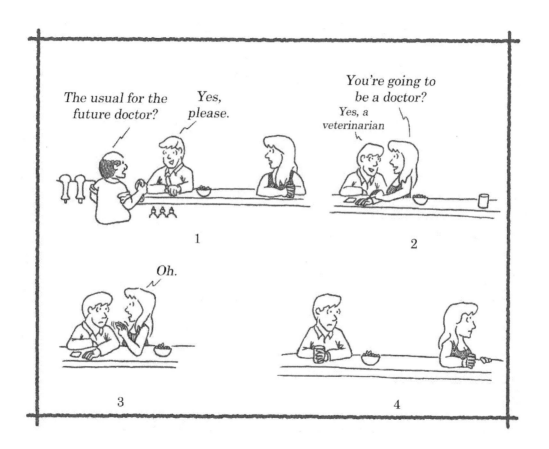

177

Not realizing your rectal glove was torn
until you itch you nose three hours later.

Confusing the os penis with a
foreign body on a radiograph.

Examining a cow with a vestibule bigger
than your $600/month studio apartment.

Realizing during parasitology that those haven't been
rice kernels in your feces for the last seven years.

Pithing an animal during your first attempt
at a jugular stick.

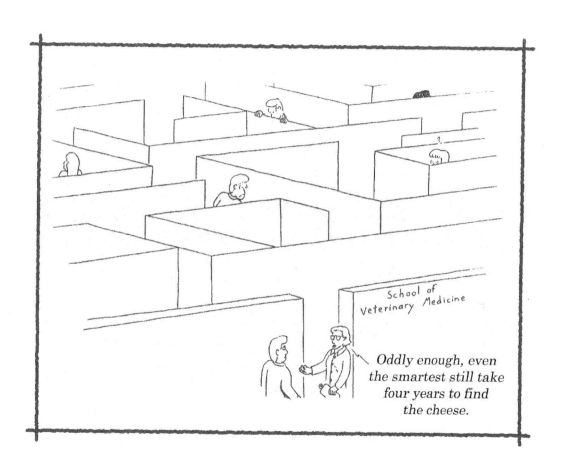

Clients seem to understand what you are
saying even if you don't.

You come to school in darkness, leave home in
darkness, and spend all day in a haze.

You can't decide whether to use one-handed or
two-handed ties to close your sneakers.

After ten exams in as many weeks,
you find you've lost your menace reflex.

Your sneaker laces dehisce.

Interpreting Expressions
During Surgery

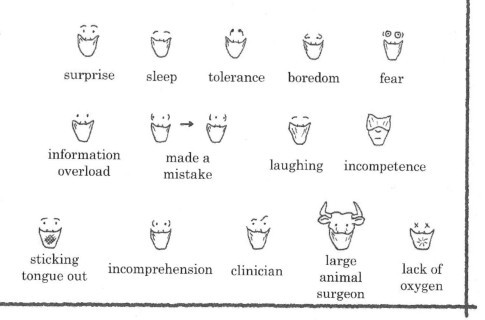

surprise sleep tolerance boredom fear

information overload made a mistake laughing incompetence

sticking tongue out incomprehension clinician large animal surgeon lack of oxygen

You know you are in fourth year when you start longing for
the simple easy days of second year.

Your surgery partner, "More Aseptic Than Thou",
has taken to autoclaving her underwear.

Only after you finish the last exam of the quarter is it
revealed that the exam was accidentally put on reserve in
the library two days ago and half the class
had already seen it.

Your family asks you not to describe food
by referring to lesions.

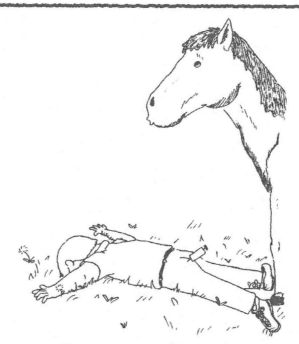

The tranquilizer meant for the horse
pierces your left buttock.

Your pathology professor informs you that you will no longer be permitted to describe lesions by referring to foods that look similar.

You wonder if the saying, "The more you learn, the more you realize how much you don't know" is true. And, if it is, then with all that you don't know, why aren't you the smartest person in school?

While juggling your hepatic encephalopathy, diabetes mellitus, and recovering GDV cases, you hear about the other students who have the suspicious luck of only getting vaccination cases.

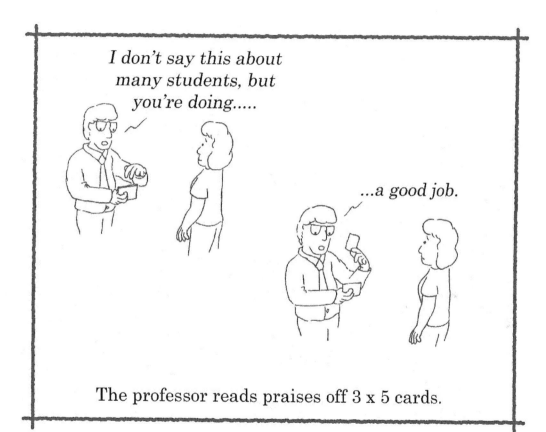

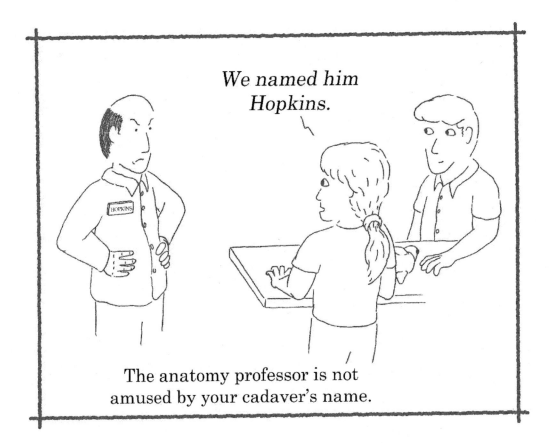

You realize that some of your classmates will be the same age at graduation that you were when you entered veterinary school.

There's a new prescription diet for the nutritional management of less-active veterinary students. It's by Hills and called v/d.

You become a pawn in a power-struggle involving the senior radiology technician, his least favorite clinician, and an incontinent greyhound.

Your remote control from home doesn't work on the TV or DVD players in the surgery tape viewing room.

The First Row
(as seen by the second row)

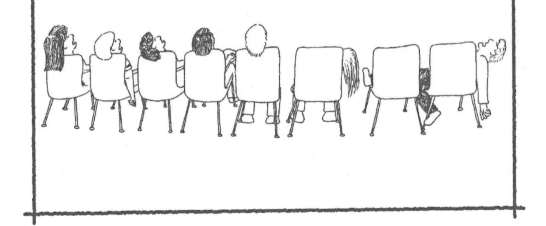

You set your alarm clock wrong and it doesn't
wake you at the end of class.

Life as a truck driver is starting to look like a viable option.

A fourth-year requirement is to put your first-year
anatomy cadaver back together.

You're disappointed to find out that
Current Veterinary Therapy
is <u>not</u> a mental health book.

The faculty reveal that, sometimes, when they're not sure,
they just make stuff up to see if you notice.

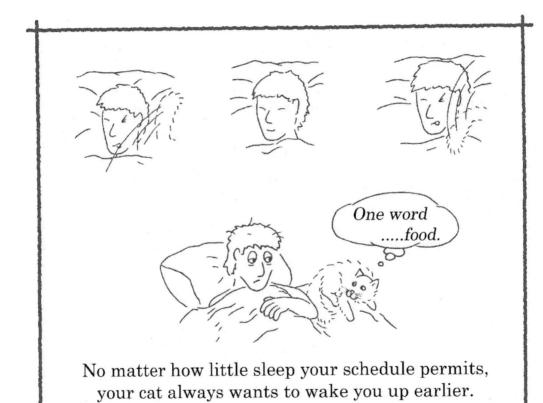

No matter how little sleep your schedule permits,
your cat always wants to wake you up earlier.

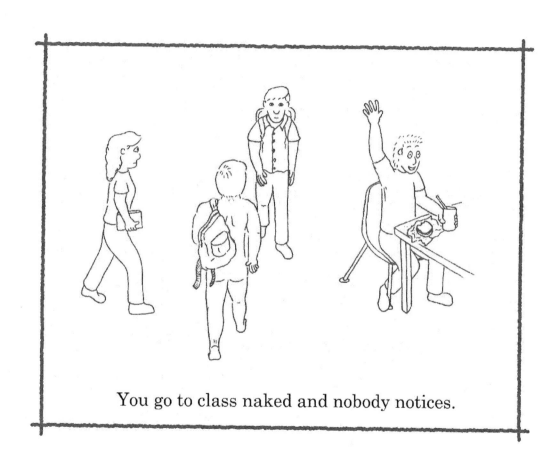

You go to class naked and nobody notices.

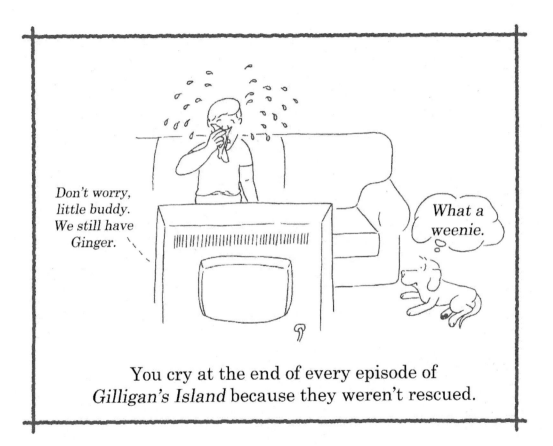

You cry at the end of every episode of
Gilligan's Island because they weren't rescued.

Your half-life for information-retention is about 20 seconds
which is why you have to take such frequent doses.

You have a recurring dream of surgeons peering down
at you saying, "Since this is our first surgery,
it'll be non-survival, right?"

You fall in love, fall out of love, fall in love, fall out of love,
fall in love, fall out of love.....then you graduate.

Two A.M. on Easter Sunday, the
Easter Bunny's hidden a colored egg
in the proximal duodenum of your dog.

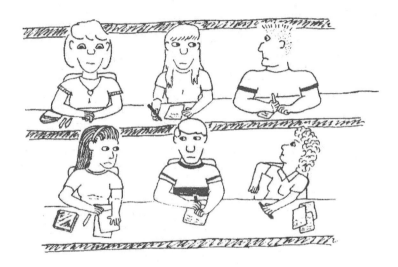

Being in a class of 100 people and not
being able to figure out who just farted.

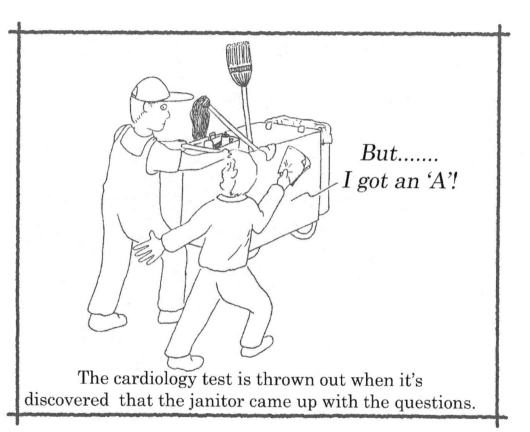

The cardiology test is thrown out when it's discovered that the janitor came up with the questions.

*Anyone who doesn't return their microscope
spends a night in the box! Anyone talking in
class spends a night in the box! Anyone needing
to go to the bathroom during class spends a
night in the box. Anyone asking
silly questions.....*

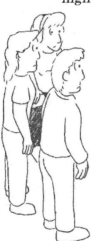
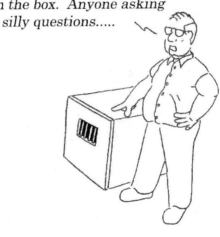

The vet school's rules seem a little restrictive.

Professors who hum the song *"Live and Let Die"*
while you take their exams.

An hour into the reading material it dawns on you
that you've already read this once before.

You've learned more about your fellow
classmates than you ever wanted to know.

Part of your registration packet is to take
out a life insurance policy.

Finding out that a dental hygienist
makes more than a veterinarian.

THE REGENTS OF THE

University of California

ON THE NOMINATION OF THE FACULTY OF THE SCHOOL OF VETERINARY MEDICINE

HAVE CONFERRED UPON

DEAN W. SCOTT

THE DEGREE OF DOCTOR OF VETERINARY MEDICINE

WITH ALL THE RIGHTS AND PRIVILEGES THERETO PERTAINING

GIVEN AT DAVIS THIS EIGHTEENTH DAY OF JUNE IN THE YEAR

NINETEEN HUNDRED AND NINETY-THREE

GOVERNOR OF CALIFORNIA AND
PRESIDENT OF THE REGENTS

PRESIDENT OF THE UNIVERSITY

CHANCELLOR AT DAVIS

DEAN OF THE SCHOOL

Expires: 18 Jun 2013

Your diploma has an expiration date.

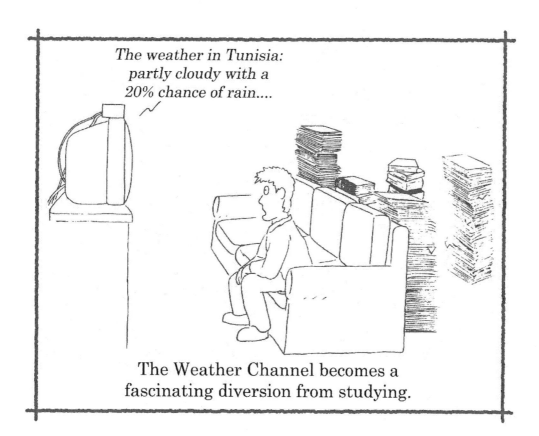

The textbook is useless except for squishing
exceptionally hard-to-kill roaches.

In vet school, the syllabus is more
important than you are.

It's become difficult to tell the difference between falling
asleep in class and going into a coma.

Class discussions are decoys to lure
you away from potential exam material.

Your courses are very thorough; what isn't covered
in class is covered on the final exam.

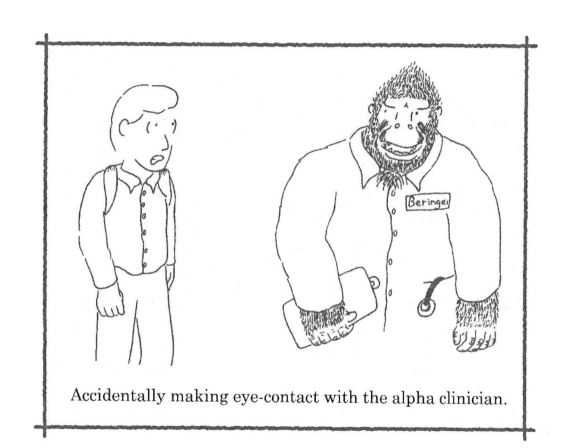

Accidentally making eye-contact with the alpha clinician.

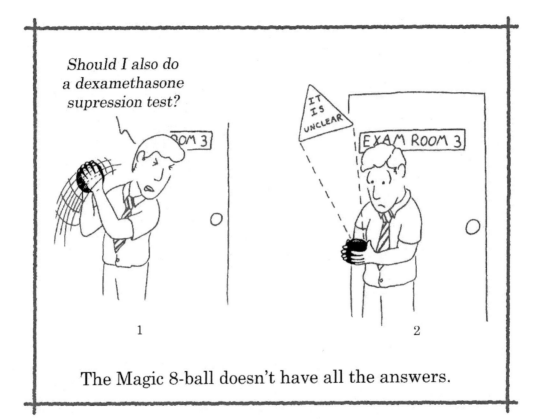

The Magic 8-ball doesn't have all the answers.

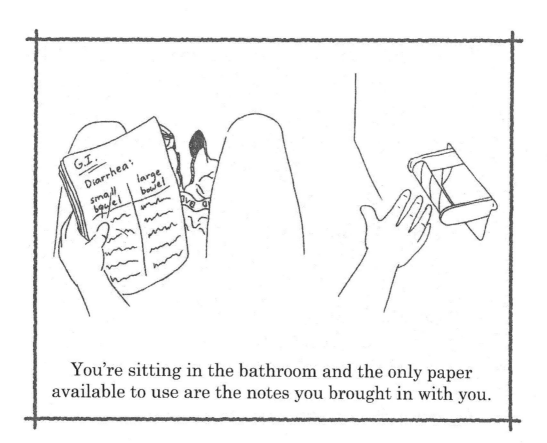

You're sitting in the bathroom and the only paper available to use are the notes you brought in with you.

You uncover a moral dilemma when, in a drunken stupor,
you score the highest grade on an exam.

You walk away after washing the dishes
with your hands in the air.

You look deep into your lover's eyes
and pull out a penlight.

You study at stop lights, during meals, on the toilet, while
brushing your teeth, while on the phone,
and during sex.

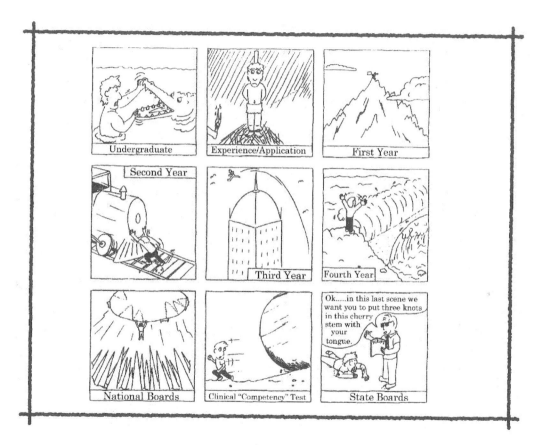

Though the bottles are very similar, you find out that there is a fundamental difference between eye lubricant and surgical glue.

You notice the hospital pager you were assigned is set on "STUN".

At graduation, a man tells you, "You may have your diploma when you can snatch the pea from my hand."

Due to a disturbance in the space-time continuum, you receive your National Board scores before you take them and........you didn't do very well.

Viewing elephant reproduction videos that turn you
off sex for months afterwards.

Being told by a clinician that it's wrong
to tell a client to put up or shut up.

Psychosis sets in due to the lack of sleep
and that's.........okay.

You've actually spent time looking up words and medical
accuracies found in the texts
and cartoons of this book.

You call your voice-mail from your car while driving
to school to remind yourself of all the tasks
you need to finish after school.

The first time you have to use your student health
insurance, you find that they won't cover anything.

Having to explain to the professor that yes, indeed, your
dog did chew up your homework.

Finding you can quote all the previous stresses
without referring to the list.

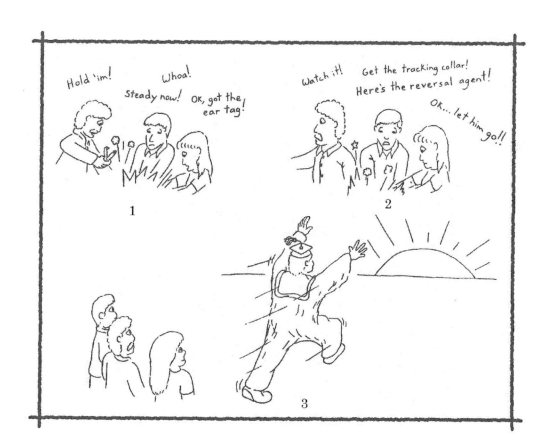

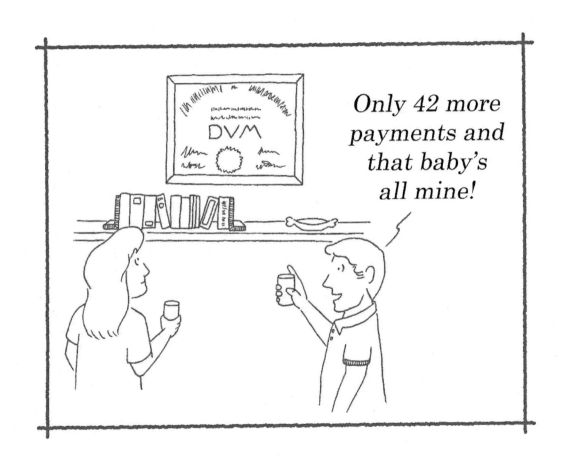

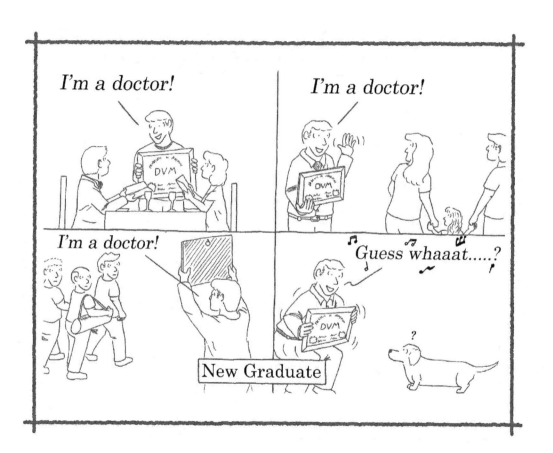

Final Thoughts

There are plenty of places you can go to get help about how to study efficiently, how to takes tests, etc. The nuts and bolts of schooling. However, unless you've been through the vet school process, there is truly no way to prepare someone adequately for the grueling, grinding, unrelenting, unsympathetic nature of it. However, assuming you're masochistic enough to join this dysfunctional tribe, and I'm assuming you are because you're holding this book in your hands, let me pass on some small advice to make your life easier.

You can only do your best. And that's good enough. There will be times that you doubt this. A little doubt is okay; it keeps you attentive and learning. However, you should never doubt that you are not capable and competent. Everyone has their strengths and weaknesses. You will not be amazing and fantastic at everything. You are human. You will push yourself to be perfect and that is not a reasonable or sustainable goal. No one is perfect. If you've done your best, that's all you, or anyone else can expect. You can't do someone else's best; if you could, then you would be them. You can only do _your_ best. And other people, also, can't do what you do so well.

Don't let other people put you down. Others will almost certainly dismiss you and be condescending at one point or another. You have achieved more than most people just by getting to where you are. Just make sure you remember the skills, intelligence and tenacity it took to get you to your goals. Also, you will come across people that seem to get through effortlessly. Trust me, they are dealing with their own feelings of inadequacy and uncertainty. While it is worthwhile to push yourself, don't do it to the exclusion of everything else. Veterinary medicine is a marathon, not a sprint. You want to be in it for the long-haul.

Take care of yourself. As much as vet school (and the profession in general) tries to wear you down with the sheer amount of material and demands, take time for yourself to do something else, to decompress. Life-balance, as cliched as that sounds, is essential, not only in school, but once you graduate. Pre-vet prep geared us into hyper-drive because we were living only to get into vet school. Having achieved the goal, we continue to try to operate at that same high level. Believe it or not, it will benefit you most in the long-run to ratchet that instinct down. You will be tempted to continue to excel in every way and check-box off every activity and medical discipline. However, vet school, if you pay attention, will teach you your limits as well. We all have our limits and it's okay to acknowledge them. The best way I can phrase it is, if I could get through it, and trust me I was not a stellar student, so can you. Understand that grades alone don't make a veterinarian. Once you graduate, no one will ever ask you what your grades were.

Finally, don't take things too seriously. If I can offer nothing else, I wish to offer you permission to laugh at things, even yourself. This profession suffers too much from Seriouscytosis (which is a word I just made up). And I think that can be draining. Whether you see it in your colleagues or not, you are all under-going your own set of stressors, both external and self-inflicted. No one has it easy and we should make sure we are there for one another. The main reason for this book is to lay these stresses out, to share in their commonality, and to find something, anything, humorous about it all. You are not going through this alone, no matter how it might feel like it at times. If nothing else, I'm there with you, if only in spirit through this book. I hope it makes your vet school experience even a little bit lighter. Good luck!

Addendum1: This book would not be complete without mentioning my classmate, Sophia Yin, who was kind enough to give my material its first break and introduction to veterinary students. I can't say I knew her well, but I am forever indebted to her for going out on a limb when she was first starting her Cattledog Publishing company. She also certainly contributed even more to the veterinary community as a whole with all of her work and insights. I'm sorry she is not around to see and continue what she started and supported. One of the reasons I continue to do what I'm doing is _because_ she isn't with us anymore and I'd like to see the pressures of this profession lessen for everyone.

Addendum 2: In case, you're feeling cheated and you counted the number of stresses listed in this book and found there weren't 1,000 (and I know some of you did), that's because it takes two books to do all of this right. The other book is called *Vet Med Spread* and can be found on my website: www.funnyvet.com. I've also allowed that you will be able to round out the thousand stresses with your own, personal entries. Who knows, maybe there are even more than that. After all, we like nothing better than taking on more stresses!

Check out my website: FunnyVet. It's free. Which is exactly the right amount for an aspiring veterinarian. You'll find over 1,500 cartoons, song parodies, client comments, veterinary truisms, and a sporadically-written (hopefully humorous) blog.

Also, if you go to YouTube and type in funnyvetdotcom all as one word, you will discover more humorous videos and song parodies. Finally (honest, this is it), there's our www.cafepress.com/funnyvet page where you can find veterinary and animal-related designs to put on coffee mugs, t-shirts, mousepads, etc. Great gifts for yourself and others!

29602160R00120

Made in the USA
Lexington, KY
01 February 2019